ANTIVIRAL
AROMATHERAPY

essential oils for
health & wellbeing

MAGGIE TISSERAND

weaver

This edition published in 2022
Weaver Publishing Ltd
South Devon Hs, Babbage Rd
Totnes, Devon, TQ9 5JA
www.weaver-publishing.com

British Library Cataloguing in Publication Data

A CIP catalogue record for this book is available from the British Library.

ISBN: 978-1-9163039-2-8

Front cover design: Paul Palmer-Edwards

This book is dedicated to Mother Nature

CONTENTS

Acknowlegements

I want to thank every university researcher who had the foresight to see the potential in challenging common viruses with essential oils and carrying out in vitro research with hundreds of essential oils and their component parts. These tests took place over a number of years across the globe: Canada, Germany, South Korea, Taiwan and Turkey.

And a vote of thanks to the university research teams who, since the emergence of Covid-19, have undertaken in silico research based around the in vitro antiviral essential oil results. Computational analysis of past antiviral proof together with future hypotheses in regards to the coronavirus covered different research objectives. In silico studies had varying results, but with the collective opinion 'further research needs to be conducted with essential oils as potential treatments for Covid-19.' These studies took place in Algeria, Brazil, China, Ethiopia, India, Nigeria, Pakistan and USA.

My gratitude goes to the research teams who have documented the various ways and routes by which essential oils damage bacterial and viral membranes.

This research took place in Australia, China, Italy, Germany, India, Malaysia and The Netherlands. As membrane disruption causes viral cell death quickly and effectively, this research gives credence to the term antiviral aromatherapy.

Thanks to my son James for all his help and support with the creation of *Antiviral Aromatherapy* – from beginning to end; for proofing, taking care of technical issues and cooking me delicious vegan dinners. Appreciative thanks have to go to everyone who has sent me constructive feedback on content, making *Antiviral Aromatherapy* a better book. And finally, my thanks for all the support received from – my sister Jackie, friends Lizzie Lush, Graham Love, Nancy Silverstein, Jack Allison and Mary Dalgliesh.

Introduction

I am neither a scientist nor a medically qualified person: I am a researcher-writer with six published books on the subject of aromatherapy detailing the various ways in which essential oils can be utilized, including one book highlighting the ability of some essential oils to counteract superbugs. For many years, I have firmly believed that antiviral essential oils could help people stay free of and recover from colds, flu and viruses in general. But this book is much more than my belief in aromatherapy, as my research has uncovered many scientific research papers on the testing of essential oils against viruses. Today, when people all over the world are suffering the effects of a viral pandemic, I see no merit in staying quietly in the background, when all I have wanted to do since first hearing news about Covid-19 was to let people know that we have antiviral essential oils – and that they are readily available. So, I am not holding back and love it or hate it – this is my offering.

Historically, I have collaborated with a team of university microbiologists in a South East of England university. From that partnership, I have first-hand evidence of the power of essential oils to kill antimicrobial-resistant bacteria, with that research resulting in a published paper. A considerable amount of university research has taken place worldwide with essential oils and bacteria, but very little work has been conducted with viruses until recent years.

In 2020, when I was listening to daily news updates on the devastation caused by the new coronavirus, I found myself crying every evening in front of my television. I was desperately sad to hear that there was nothing available from the world's pharmaceutical companies to prevent or reduce the number of deaths. Nothing capable of halting the spread of the coronavirus that was ravaging nursing homes, filling hospital ICU wards. A virus that was killing large numbers of elderly people as well as younger people with underlying health conditions. I was also frustrated, as I know from experience that many essential oils are antiviral. And that two commonly available essential oils had saved the life of my infant son in the 1970s. I thought back to when a paediatric hospital doctor informed me that my son had a severe herpes simplex infection, that there were no antivirals to give him, and that it would be up to him to fight for survival. That was more than forty years ago.

Yet, in 2020, there didn't seem to have been any linear progression regarding antiviral pharmacology, and that a diagnosis of Covid-19 appeared to have an identical prognosis to the one I received in regards to my son's viral infection – the need for a person's immune system to fight for survival. There are no specific antivirals for Covid-19, although some repurposed drugs are becoming authorized for treating the most vulnerable. The rest of us will continue to fight off the virus – with or without vaccines. Most people infected with Covid-19 will recover, but there is an increased risk of mortality for anyone with a severe underlying health condition, people with an auto-immune disease, and anyone else taking immunosuppressants – as well as the elderly. Also vulnerable are the many people undergoing or recovering from chemotherapy treatment – as these drugs decimate the immune system, and my eldest daughter would have been one more 'vulnerable person' had she survived her cancer.

My personal story in PART 1 became the impetus for me to write this book, and in 2021, I became motivated to seek out research papers from universities dotted around the world and soon found evidence that essential oil research with the influenza A virus – responsible for several major flu outbreaks, including the 1918 flu pandemic – had been conducted in a South Korean university, with a scientific paper published in 2018. Over 60 essential oils had been tested, with eleven proven to be virucidal. Delighted to find this antiviral evidence, I continued my quest to find, read and digest further studies to substantiate the Seoul research. I found many published papers on the fascinating subject of 'natural antivirals'. Although they were all of interest, my focus was solely on finding documented evidence of antiviral research with essential oils. In vitro research citations led me to find an exciting new development - computational research (referred to as in silico analysis) that postulates the ability of antiviral essential oils to be further researched to aid the fight against Covid-19. Even more thrilling was finding evidence of how some essential oils can disrupt viral membranes, causing death of the virus. All of this research is available in

PART 4 of my book. I have tried to keep it simple for easy reading, but for anyone interested in further details, every research paper is fully detailed in my Citation section.

Antiviral Aromatherapy became my passion, and in writing and publishing this book, I hope it will be of some help. It is a book in four parts, and I begin, in PART 1, with anecdotal stories - my personal experience of essential oils defeating viruses. Included in that section are details of two common essential oils that I made into aromatic waters and used in the paediatric ward where my son was fighting for his life: for cleansing, disinfecting, reducing my son's high fever, and as an added bonus, to gently scent the partitioned room where my son and I lived for two weeks. Also included in PART 1 are details of a massage trial that I called 'The Nurses Stress Project', set up in 1994 and run within the main hospital in Brighton, South East England. Fifty nurses were recruited, each to receive a 45-minute massage, once a week for a period of eight weeks – completely free of charge. The project was a great success with positive and enthusiastic feedback. Today, our nurses and doctors need more than applause, more than hand sanitizers and sterile protective items – they need actual, physical support to help their immune systems repair. They need protection from the harmful, accumulative effects of working long hours with a constant flow of very sick patients suffering the ravages of coronavirus.

Essential oils can be both antibacterial and antiviral, as Mother Nature doesn't discriminate. Over decades of laboratory trials, much evidence has been accrued to prove that some essential oils are antibacterial. Only in recent years has focus switched to investigating the use of essential oils and their components for the potential of being used against viruses: influenza A and herpes simplex HSV-1 being the two most frequently tested viruses. And of great significance is the more obscure research, conducted by a small number of scientists who set up in vitro trials to examine ways in which antiviral essential oils were able to damage bacterial cell walls and viral membranes.

Essential oils, the backbone of aromatherapy, have been a big part of my life since the early 1970s, when alternative medicine was known as 'fringe medicine'.

No longer on the fringe, aromatherapy and many other alternative therapies are being used within hospital and clinical settings, although mainly in palliative care. Not all essential oils are equal, and in PART 2, I have referred to twenty-one essential oils that have been proven antiviral in university trials. A brief write up from each paper can be found in PART 4, with full citations in the following Citations section. PART 2 also contains a comprehensive overview of aromatherapy. What are essential oils? How to use essential oils and when to be cautious. The process from raw plant material to a bottle of essential oil, the importance of understanding how concentrated they are, and why we need to respect them. Over many decades of using essential oils, I have learned which ones work on the body, the brain and the emotions, and this gives me the confidence to say that every essential oil mentioned in *Antiviral Aromatherapy* could, in one way or another, help to relieve the symptoms of long Covid.

I have been following clues – like an amateur detective – scanning the citations of each published paper, moving ever forward to find as many university papers as possible and then to choose the most relevant.

Now, in this time of viral illness, I want to introduce the world to antiviral essential oils. It could be said that Mother Nature is responsible for the coronavirus – and we may wonder why – but when I think back to my childhood and the pain and discomfort inflicted by stinging nettles followed by the instant relief from rubbing dock leaves over the affected area, I am full of respect for the close proximity of the antidote. That is why, in PART 4 of this book, you will find a summary of ten in vitro research papers, eight in silico research papers; and ten papers detailing the membrane disrupting capabilities of a small selection of essential oils. I am repeating myself somewhat, as not all readers will wish to read PART 4 of my book as it is pretty academic, and I want everyone to know that this book contains indisputable facts about several virucidal essential oils. They are safe to use, are inexpensively priced, and are on sale in your neighbourhood.

The hard facts are that we live in a world of uncertainty, where the availability of vaccines is tempering fear and a sense of disempowerment, but where we have no cures and no medical preventatives. Regarding general advice on ways of staying well, there is advice on handwashing, mask-wearing and social distancing. But where is the education and encouragement to support and protect our immune system – so that it can be at its most effective? PART 3 is all about the immune system, but as it seems that we know more about the solar system than the immune system, I have gathered together important information together with a lot of facts and figures and then included my simple calculations as to the speed at which viruses multiply and why immediate action could save lives. Although pharmaceutical companies may be in the process of researching new drugs to kill the coronavirus – without harming human beings – the journey from laboratory to pharmacy shelves is long and arduous. So, while we are waiting for Big Pharma drugs and government approvals, I have written and published this book: *to divulge what I know about essential oils, the immune system and the available scientific evidence.* Of the hundreds of essential oils on sale and the many tested, I have listed twenty-one antiviral essential oil in PART 2. I want it to be known that there is an alternative to 'waiting and hoping' and that we all have the option to be proactive in our health and wellbeing by making good use of what the natural world has already provided.

ANTIVIRAL AROMATHERAPY

PART 1
ANTIVIRAL ESSENTIAL OILS – IN ACTION

Aromatherapy has been a big part of my life for more than forty years, and my love and respect for essential oils only gets stronger over time. Essential oils are my go-to remedies whenever I feel under attack from germs – viral, bacterial, fungal. Essential oils don't discriminate; they simply work with the immune system to deal with invading pathogens. Over the years of successfully remaining clear of my doctor's consulting room, my strategy has always been and will always be to 'nip it in the bud' rather than wait for a disease to become 'full-blown'. Preventative medicine makes perfect sense to me and is the reason why I have written this book. Below are a few examples of the powerful ways in which essential oils work with the immune system to fight off a virus and restore health and wellbeing.

How my infant son survived a severe viral infection

"Your son has herpes simplex virus and is very poorly. I'm sorry to have to tell you that we don't have any medicine to give him. It's up to your son to fight this if he is going to survive." The doctor walked out of the glass-walled cubicle of the paediatric ward in a north London hospital, and I burst into tears. I thought that my son was going to die. He was just fifteen months old. Without any pharmaceutical intervention to counteract the virus and fearing for my son's life, it seemed almost miraculous that he was free of the virus and discharged from the hospital just over two weeks later. He had recovered from a severe infection of herpes simplex that had overwhelmed his body's defences. His primary nurse was me, and the healing medicine had been a few drops of lavender oil and eucalyptus oil, each used in a particular way. Back in 1975, I never imagined that one day these two essential oils would be scientifically proven to be antiviral – see PART 4 – although I was aware of their historical reputation for being antiseptic and able to lower a high body temperature.

Above is the short version of an anecdotal story taken from my first book, *Aromatherapy for Women* – below is the long version.

In late 1975, my one-year-old son was desperately ill. As we were subsequently to discover, he was highly allergic to dairy products. He was hospitalised for tests to determine what was wrong with him. Back then, the paediatric doctor – and it would seem at that time, the entire medical profession – believed that a baby could not be allergic to cows' milk, even though I had explained several times that my son had been perfectly healthy prior to the introduction of baby food containing dried milk powder. At some stage during the five-week hospital stay and following many tests, I was invited to speak with the paediatrician in his office, and on walking in, heard the words, "We can't find what is wrong with your son. We have run all the tests we can: breast milk is satisfactory but is no longer being produced in sufficient quantity. We are at a complete loss." Hearing this statement gave me the courage to speak assertively – "You don't believe me when I tell you that my son is allergic to cows' milk, so get some milk, now, and give it to him. You need to see for yourself." Instructions were given for a pint of milk to be fetched from the nurses' kitchen, and I watched as the doctor poured a small amount onto a spoon and put a little into my son's mouth. Instantaneously, blisters appeared on his lips.

The doctor gasped and uttered the words, "Oh, my dear, you were right all along; your son has just displayed a severe allergic reaction." From that moment on, the doctor did his utmost to swiftly procure a supply of soya bean infant formula, which had to be flown in from the USA, as there was no vegan milk formula available in the UK. My son thrived on the soy formula and soon gained weight. It was a five-week progression from admission to discharge: today the progress would be swift as food allergies and intolerances are now well documented.

A few months later, I thought my son would benefit from interaction with other children, so I took him to a mother and toddler group. At the time, I did not have much understanding of immunity and how my son's milk allergy and subsequent lack of protein had seriously depleted his immune system. One of the other toddlers had a runny nose but was otherwise fine. Within a few days, my son became extremely ill. Instead of developing a cold, as one would have expected, he developed severe herpes simplex, with pustular lesions inside his mouth and a lesion in one of his eyes. His weakened immune system had been overwhelmed, and what had been 'a runny nose' for one child had become a 'life-threatening disease' for mine.

And once again, my son was admitted to the hospital, where the paediatric doctor informed me that as it was a viral infection and there was no medicine available to help, he would have to fight it off himself to survive. Thankfully, I was allowed to stay in my son's cubicle, sleeping overnight on a fold-out camp bed next to his cot. Over the next few days, my son's temperature increased, and of great concern to me was witnessing a discharge of pustular matter from the lesions inside his mouth. I used disposable nappies, placing a fresh one under his face every few hours to absorb the discharge. I swabbed the inside of his mouth with very diluted, luke-warm lavender water, continuing this regime for several days. When his temperature rose unacceptably high, I used a eucalyptus foot compress to reduce the fever. Eucalyptus is a well-known febrifuge (something to reduce fever). I used a clean dishcloth from the ward kitchen, dipped it into the eucalyptus water, and after wringing out the cloth, wrapped it around my son's feet.

When the cloth dried out, I repeated the procedure, and by touching my son's forehead and body, I was able to tell that his temperature was reducing. As he became more comfortable, the grizzling stopped, and he fell asleep. That's when I slid into my sleeping bag on the camp bed and slept until 2 a.m. when the night nurse entered for a scheduled temperature check. I felt confident in declining the intervention as my son no longer had a fever and was sleeping peacefully – but I had to sign a disclaimer before getting back into bed. I had been my son's primary nurse, and by diligently utilising two essential oils, the virus had been defeated. In less than two weeks, the worst of the crisis was over, and my son was able to drink from a bottle once more, instead of being fed via a nasal-stomach tube. The lavender water had cleansed, disinfected, and healed the herpes lesions in the mouth; the eucalyptus water had reduced his temperature, and I was able to take my son home. Looking back on my actions, following what had seemed to be a 'death sentence' from the paediatric doctor, I am proud to say that I did not give in to the pronouncement "We don't have anything to help your son." 'We', in the 1970s, was the paediatric ward of a north London hospital, and quite possibly the entirety of the UK medical profession, but I did not give in to fear and hopelessness. Sitting and hoping for the best was not for me. I needed to be proactive and try my very best to help my son fight the virus. And with nothing more than a heart full of love and two essential oils, my son recovered from a severe viral infection that could easily have taken his life.

Neonatal herpes is a viral infection in a young baby. The younger the baby, the more vulnerable they are to the harmful effects of the virus. Herpes can be very serious for a young baby whose immune system is not sufficiently developed to fight off the virus. It can also be serious for a toddler with a damaged immune system. Because newborn babies have underdeveloped immune systems, they can quickly become very ill after catching the virus. The main symptoms are: high fever and sores on the skin, eyes and inside the mouth. Nowadays, neonatal herpes is treated with intravenous antiviral drugs, which might be required for several weeks. When neonatal herpes only affects the baby's eyes, mouth or skin, most babies will make a complete recovery with antiviral treatment. Still, the condition is much more dangerous if it has spread to the baby's internal organs, and almost a third of infants with systemic neonatal herpes will die, even after intravenous treatment.

Simple to make aromatic waters

Eucalyptus water for a foot compress to reduce fever
You will need a clean glass jar with a screw-on lid filled halfway with water. Count out one or two drops of eucalyptus essential oil – depending on the jar size and amount of water – 1 drop of eucalyptus for a small jar, two drops for a larger size. Screw on the lid, and shake the jar vigorously to disperse the eucalyptus oil throughout the water. Pour the liquid into a bowl and immediately dip in a cloth of a good size for the area to be treated. For tiny feet – like my child's – a small washcloth was perfect. Adult feet would require larger cloths such as hand towels or dish-drying cloths – one for wrapping around each foot. Remove the cloths when dry and repeat the procedure. Bear in mind that essential oils do not dissolve in water, and for this reason, it is necessary to shake the jar of liquid vigorously

and use it immediately; otherwise, the essential oil will separate from the water and float on top.

Lavender water for cleansing a baby's mouth and lips
I used very dilute lavender water to cleanse the inside of my son's cheeks and also clean his lips. To a small glass jar, half-filled with water, I added one drop of lavender essential oil, and with the lid screwed on tight, the jar was vigorously shaken. I used cotton wool balls that were soft and small yet firm enough to wipe the inside of a baby's mouth and lips. I always had a small plastic bag nearby so that each cotton ball could be hygienically contained and easily disposable. This procedure needed to be repeated many times in a 24hr period, as the herpes virus infection was life-threatening. The actions I performed were like those of an intensive care nurse, but with alterative medicine.

Herpes simplex, the common cold, influenza and antiviral essential oils – my story
In my mid-thirties, I first became infected with the herpes simplex virus, with hot, sore blisters on my lips that reappeared every time I became stressed. Stress was a frequent occurrence for me as a single mother

of three children, and taking care of everything involved with schools, running a household, writing books and generally juggling and struggling to keep a roof over our heads during the early post-divorce years. It is a medical fact that herpes simplex does not go away but lives in the central nervous system, and when the body is under stress, the virus re-emerges. The virus is known as 'persistent', and once infected, you are infected for life. I believed that to be the case, but over the years of using essential oils at the first sign of infection and taking care of sore throats and coughs at the earliest opportunity, I have become more resistant to outbreaks of herpes simplex. Even while coping with incredibly stressful life events – and nowadays a cold sore is a very rare occurrence. Several antiviral essential oils are suitable for treating a cold sore – tea tree, lemon, and melissa are the main oils I used over the years, and found that any one of them would work quickly to relieve the itching and swelling. Clove oil also works well, although it stings a little.

Winter colds and influenza viruses are also 'historical events' for me as I have for many decades incorporated tiny amounts of essential oils into my lifestyle – but always used with respect as essential oils are concentrated and should not be overused. The outcome is that I have not suffered from a cold in over ten years, and it's been more than five decades since I was ill with influenza. I clearly remember the last time I suffered from influenza as I was nineteen years old and had only recently left home for a more independent life. I recovered very quickly from the flu after a friend recommended I buy a bottle of concentrated essence of cinnamon – not an essential oil, but an extract from the cinnamon tree. I bought a bottle, and it worked! It is available online to this day.

The above stories are about individuals – but the following story is about fifty nurses: each one an individual, yet sharing the same stressors – a heavy workload, sleep disturbance from shift work, being close to distressed patients daily, every working day confined to a germ-laden environment, and for many, the added stresses of juggling finances in order to get by. The following story is about a project I conceived in 1994, set up, financed and project-managed – with permission from the Royal Sussex Hospital Trust and with free use of hospital facilities.

The Nurses Stress Project

Research has been conducted into the sleeping capability of nurses whose sleep patterns are interrupted regularly. Results of this research indicate that a high proportion of nurses experience difficulty in sleeping soundly, as they can't get into a regular sleep-wake cycle. In general, nurses are contracted to work eight-hour rotating shifts: 8 a.m – 4 p.m; 4 p.m – midnight; midnight to 8 a.m. This kind of stress can cause a myriad of health problems.

I ran an eight-week trial in Brighton to see whether nursing staff would benefit from having a weekly aromatherapy massage. With permission from the CEO of the hospital trust and free use of a daytime-only clinic for five evenings a week over eight weeks, I pulled together a team of volunteers from a massage training school. Twenty newly qualified massage therapists donated their time to the trial, with only their out-of-pocket expenses covered. I also persuaded a friend to manage the evening project and called it 'The Nurses Stress Project.' This account was included in my book *Stress: The Aromatic Solution*, published in 1996.

The Nurses Stress Project involved the recruiting of fifty nurses, as that was a manageable number for the newly trained therapists. It was relatively easy to bring the therapists on board, but I wasn't sure how to attract nurses. A member of the hospital management suggested that I pin a message to the notice board in the corridor outside the staff restaurant. The offer of a weekly 45-minute massage, over an eight-week period, was taken up very quickly and soon over-subscribed – with a waiting list for any spare time slots. Many of the nurses had never experienced a massage before. However, some were familiar with aromatherapy or had come into contact with the use of essential oils within a hospital ward.

Before the massage treatment began, each nurse filled in a questionnaire detailing their stress levels, sleep patterns and other minor health issues. Each treatment consisted of a simple back and neck massage with one of three pre-blended massage oils that I had formulated. One blend was an energising mixture for those nurses who stated that they were 'tired all the time'. Another blend contained essential oils known to be uplifting and soothing for nurses who were stressed or depressed. The final blend consisted of essential oils that are known to fight infection and strengthen the immune system, and this was used for nurses who said they 'always had a sore throat'. From the third week onwards, each nurse could choose the blend she wanted – according to how she had responded to the initial two massage sessions.

At the end of week one, the questionnaires had revealed that 62% of nurses felt that their stress levels were moderate, whilst 32% stated that their stress levels were fairly high to very high, accompanied by a range of un-well symptoms. Most commonly, the un-wellness was 'a permanently sore throat' and 'chronic insomnia'. To one degree or another, common to every nurse was a raft of physical ailments that included backache, tense shoulders and a sore neck, which worsened whenever the lifting of a heavy weight became necessary. Overall, it was clear from the questionnaires that almost all of the fifty nurses were suffering from neck and shoulder tension, combined with a chronic lack of sleep. Some nurses admitted that feeling 'not quite well' on a regular basis caused irritability, oversensitivity, and depression.

After only two or three massage sessions, some of the nurses were experiencing a reduction of pain in their necks, shoulders, and backs. Sleep levels were vastly improved, with one nurse reporting that, instead of the two to four hours she was used to, she was now sleeping for six hours or more. Another nurse who had regularly suffered from a sore throat for six days out of every seven, was surprised to find that her throat was only sore for one or two days a week during her third week of treatment. Overall, the trial was a great success, and the only negative feedback came from a few male nurses, who complained that they too suffered from stress and sleep problems and felt aggrieved that they had not been invited onto the trial. It was my decision to run the initial trial as female nurses only.

Here are a few unsolicited comments from some of the nurses:

"I found it hard to believe how much stress affects our bodies until I had my shoulders and neck massage. They have never felt so good in ten years as a nurse."

"I found that the raised energy levels, better sleep and fewer infections all ended when the massage trial came to an end."

"I had been experiencing sleep disturbance for some time. However, the night of the sessions, I certainly slept better and felt relaxed."

"I felt really laid back, and little things didn't irritate me so much. I found I learned to relax."

One nurse summed up the general feeling amongst the fifty nurses taking part in the 8-week trial – "I cannot thank you all enough for helping to improve my physical and psychological well-being."

The fact that the trial was a 'one-off' saddened some nurses who thought it should be an integral part of hospital life.

Although I had been involved with aromatherapy for more than twenty years and believe in it wholeheartedly, even I was surprised by the enthusiasm shown by the nurses when only a quarter of the way through the trial, the majority of nurses taking part had experienced tangible benefits. Some were even discussing the feasibility of having regular aromatherapy massage sessions incorporated into hospital life as previously mentioned. Sadly, the NHS always seems to have financial struggles, and the idea was unfeasible. Yet it could be achieved privately, and I stand by the saying 'where there is a will, there is a way'. What I managed to accomplish with 50 nurses in 1994 could be made to happen on a grand scale – now, in the second decade of the twenty-first century, in the midst of a pandemic!

I think that the current hospital situation, with waves of coronavirus cases, nursing staff working until exhausted – some even losing their lives – has brought to public attention the need for a hospital system that values and supports the health and wellbeing of every nurse, every doctor and all of the individuals who form part of the hospital team. Collectively, they are like society's immune system: rushing to help the next person, and the next person, and the next person; mobilising and coordinating skills, equipment, medication, surgeries, vehicles, ancillary staff – and so much more. Nervous energy is only meant to be used in times of emergency and is not meant to be part of everyday living. Yet, in this time of Covid-19, nurses and doctors and other care workers are living on nervous energy as part of their daily lives.

In my idealistic imagination, there needs to be a nursing reserve force, just as the army has a reserve force. They would not be in a position of authority but under supervision; extra pairs of hands when needed. To be there to help turn a patient, to change bedding, to help feed someone, to hold the hand of a person nearing death – and so much more. The coronavirus pandemic is highlighting what is important in the world: and in hospitals, it is apparent that we as a society cannot 'do without' medical care; a comforting presence when medicine can't save lives. Might a more altruistic approach be a preventative measure that could halt the tide of nurses' resignations? I find it very sad that the very people we rely on to serve us in our time of need are themselves suffering from immune deficiency. How can we continue to let this happen?

Being realistic, I understand that the NHS is constantly struggling with finances, and it could be a very long time

– or never – before a 'nurses stress project' is implemented. What is needed, right now, is one or two philanthropists to fund an initiative, get it set up quickly in one area of the country, and then roll it out at a comfortable pace across the whole country. I can't see any other way for nursing staff to get the physical care and support they need during this unprecedented, demanding time in the midst of a viral pandemic. And I know it is possible. If I could conduct the project with fifty nurses, a dozen volunteer therapists and limited finances, it should be relatively easy for an experienced project manager backed by philanthropy to run a similar project. I have already run the pilot study – and it was a great success!

In early 2021, a paper was published in Occupational Medicine, following a 2020 study led by Professor* Neil Greenberg, King's College London – stating that approximately half of ICU staff had suffered such severe levels of stress that they met the threshold for PTSD. Post Traumatic Stress Disorder is generally associated with military veterans after leaving a war zone and once back home, trying to cope with their physical, mental and emotional trauma, often with nothing more than alcohol and antidepressants, which don't cure the problem.

PTSD in nursing staff has been the result of working in a constantly stressful environment with the first wave of Covid-19. And it is not hard to see why. For the first time on a national level many ICU/Critical Care staff have had to deal with ethically challenging decisions because of issues such as limited availability of ventilators: along with the high rate of mortality amongst Covid-19 patients, and working with the constant fear of catching Covid-19 and passing it on to their families.

*Full details in Citations.

We are living through a challenging time, and staying healthy is one of the most important things we can do – for ourselves, for our loved ones and our nursing staff. The healthier the general population can remain, the less hospitalisation will be necessary.

PART 2
ESSENTIAL OILS AND WAYS TO USE THEM

In this section, I will cover several subjects involving the use of essential oils – it is up to you to decide what information is of interest.

Three distinct ways of using antiviral essential oils
1. As a preventative
2. First response
3. Alternative medicine

What do I mean by 'a preventative'?
I regard the use of antiviral essential oils – when vaporized into the atmosphere of a room, to be preventative, as the amount of airborne virus that is breathed in can be reduced. A virus cannot be seen with the naked eye, and the use of airborne essential oils within the home cannot be proven to work.

However, university researchers have tested and verified that certain essential oils can successfully kill airborne viruses.

What do I mean by 'first response'?

In general, a first responder is a person who attends to a critical situation ahead of the arrival of a professional response team – a doctor or paramedic. For example, if a person near you collapses with a heart attack, a first response should be CPR after calling for an ambulance. Cardiopulmonary resuscitation is a lifesaving technique that could save more lives. And, if we should ever see a person suddenly display signs of a stroke, the immediate response should be to call for an ambulance. So in your own home, if self-isolating or beginning to feel unwell with signs of coronavirus, the prudent use of antiviral essential oils could be viewed as a 'first response'. At the first signs of a sore throat or cough, for example, a diluted blend of antiviral essential oils rubbed into the neck, collarbone, and down the sternum could prevent the virus from multiplying. Ignoring the early signs of infection is likely to allow the virus to multiply. So, while isolating and not knowing whether your next test will be positive or negative, it would be an excellent time to be inhaling antiviral essential oils. The simplest way is to add one or two drops of your chosen oil to a mug of hot water – or an electric vaporiser – and inhale the vapours. Don't wait for the virus to multiply – be your own 'first responder'.

What do I mean by 'alternative medicine'?

The use of essential oils in specific ways to treat the symptoms of long Covid could be thought of as alternative medicine – especially as there are (currently) no available pharmaceutical medicines for the symptoms of anosmia (loss of smell). As the title 'long Covid' covers a multitude of ailments that commonly follow recovery from Covid-19 infection, there are many symptoms that could be addressed by using essential oils. Further into this section, I have written a detailed account of 'treating long Covid symptoms.' Rarely are prescription medicines prescribed as cures – although there are a few exceptions. Doctors treat symptoms, matching pathology with pharmacology, hoping that the medication will clear up the health problem.

What is an essential oil?

Before we can understand how essential oils work on the body, it is necessary to understand the nature of essential oils. Although called essential oils, they are unlike fatty oils for cooking or adding to a salad. An essential oil is a non-greasy liquid. It is a unique substance, being part liquid and part volatile, for example it evaporates at room temperature. It is fragrant, and its molecules are lighter than air – therefore, it dissipates fragrance into its immediate surroundings to form a vapour that can be inhaled.

Although all essential oils evaporate into the air, they do this at different rates. Lemon essential oil, pressed from the lemon rind, is lightweight and evaporates quickly; most essential oils evaporate moderately; a few are very thick and evaporate slowly, depending on their viscosity. An essential oil is the fragrant liquid drops found within aromatic plants such as lavender and rosemary. When rubbed between the fingertips, these herbs and flowers release their hidden fragrance, as cells containing volatile oil are broken open. When not contained within a capped bottle, an essential oil will naturally diffuse into the air of a building or vehicle.

Volatile vapours are drawn in through the nose; some will reach the lungs, some will pass into the bloodstream via the lymphatic system, and others will travel through bodily organs before being eliminated.

Because essential oils are liquid and can mix with other fatty oils and liquid waxes – such as jojoba – they are known as 'lipophilic'. They are very concentrated and will always need to be diluted in a suitable base. Some people prefer to make a massage blend with fragrance-free lotion. Although a few exceptions exist, the recommended percentage of essential oils to a massage oil base is 1%–2%. Full details can be found later in this section.

Essential oils will not dissolve in water (they are hydrophobic) but can be dispersed in water – for use in several ways. When added to a full bath, the right essential oil can be trusted to gently clean wounds and skin infections. A compress with essential oils can soothe inflammation of the skin or reduce a high temperature. Aromatic waters can be made by putting one or two drops into a screw-top glass jar, half-full of water (warm or cold) and then vigorously shaking the oil/water mix. This mixture needs to be used straight away as, if left standing, the essential oil will separate from the water and float on top.

How essential oils work with the immune system

The lymphatic system is part of the immune system and is one medium through which essential oils are carried around the body. Essential oils massaged into the body will penetrate the skin, enter the bloodstream, and be moved around the body. When passing through lymph nodes they help fight infections, working directly with the immune system. Inhaled essential oil vapours travel quickly through the respiratory system to the lungs, having passed across epithelial cells where they have the opportunity of fighting a viral infection. And when essential oils are diluted in a carrier oil and massaged into the skin, they pass through many organs as they travel through the bloodstream. Whichever way they are used, essential oils are eventually eliminated from the body via the lungs, the skin, urine or faeces. The immune system does not see essential oils as a threat but a helper, as they are lipophilic. An average woman's body fat is 25%-31% and the human brain is 60% fat, so there is compatibility. It's a love affair.

Organic or non-organic

When I am faced with a viral or bacterial infection, the most crucial factor in choosing an essential oil to treat my symptoms has everything to do with the antiviral or antibacterial potency of the essential oil, and nothing to do with whether the essential oil comes from plants grown organically or traditionally. This point is especially important in the big picture of a viral pandemic, as an essential oil that works is what matters. However, organic essential oils are preferred for skincare products, although they are usually more expensive than traditionally grown essential oils.

How to choose essential oils

Essential oils are available from high street stores and through online aromatherapy essential oil suppliers. When looking for essential oil suppliers, take time to do some research. Read customer feedback and check for value for money. Compare prices and sizes – some essential oils are sold in 5ml bottles, some in 9ml or 10ml bottles, and in the USA may be sold in ounces or grams. Labels should always include volume, common name, Latin name, and country of origin and come in a tinted glass bottle.

Pure: What does that mean?

What is pure essential oil? Pure essential oil is the 100% distilled essence of an aromatic plant. Because of its concentrated form, an essential oil must be diluted before applying to the skin. Using essential oils neat on the skin can damage soft tissue, cause severe itching, long-term irritation, and make people feel sick or lethargic. Essential oils should always be used with respect. Just because something is pure does not mean that it is safe to use undiluted, and here I will try to give a personal example, even if it sounds silly.

Whenever I have flown long distances, my maximum baggage allowance has been 20 kilos, which I have found to be the maximum weight I can lift. As I get older, I struggle to lift my luggage off the trolley and onto the baggage conveyor belt. So five of those heavy 20-kilo pieces of luggage would equal 100 kilos, and if a lavender farmer harvested 100 kilos of lavender and had it distilled, he would receive one kilo of lavender oil. Not many people would be capable of picking up five 20-kilo bags, yet, with one hand, I can pick up a one-kilogram bottle of lavender oil. That is my attempt at conveying the need to respect the concentrated product of distillation. So please, remember that each essential oil is a concentrate and never let yourself be persuaded to use essential oils neat on the skin, even if someone says, "it's OK to use them neat because they are pure." That would be bad advice.

Yield: Taking lavender as an example

I'm going to take lavender as an example as I have been to the south of France and witnessed farmers bring their bundles of freshly harvested lavender to the still, where every farmer's lavender is weighed and the weight recorded against his name. A 'collective' of lavender farmers is the norm, as distillation is highly technical, requires expert knowledge, and is very expensive. Farmers throw their lavender crop into a very large receptacle – big enough for about 20 men to stand inside – then one or two men climb in and stamp down the plant material to make room for more, and this continues until the still is completely full. Then the lid is lowered into place, sealed tight, and the process of distillation begins. If a farmer has put one hundred kilos of lavender into the still, he receives one kilo of lavender oil, as that equates to a 1% yield from his 100 kilos of plant material.

Distillation

Steam distillation is the commonly used method of distillation and was once the favourite choice of lavender farmers, where plant material was placed on a metal grid until the still was fully loaded, and low-pressure steam was passed through the plant material. Nowadays, the preferred method is high-pressure steam distillation. Lavender has to be distilled within 48 hours of harvesting to achieve a good yield and as previously mentioned it takes one hundred kilos of the lavender plant to produce just one kilo of lavender oil. Whether subjected to low or high-pressure distillation, the outcome is the same – the steam dislodges the volatile plant liquid that then becomes mixed with steam. It is eventually transported through a cooler that condenses the vapour into aromatic water. The final stage is when the liquid enters a vessel known as a florentine flask, where the essential oil floats on top of the water and is easily siphoned off.

The limbic system

The only part of the brain that is open to the world is the limbic system; all other brain systems are contained safely within the skull, and as previously mentioned, I am giving the limbic system a separate section because without it, there would be no such thing as aromatherapy.

Firstly, essential oils are aromatic molecules that are inhaled via the nose; they then travel through the nasal passages to the limbic system, where the brain can identify which aroma is being inhaled. Secondly, the immune system is situated very close to the olfactory epithelium cells – and we are reliably informed that the first route of infection taken by airborne viruses is via the nose.

Stress levels, memory, blood pressure and the control of heart rate are some of the many body functions that are controlled by the limbic system: it is where the sense of smell recognises 'good' and 'bad' aromas. Olfactory nerve endings in the mucous membranes, high up inside the nose, are constantly transmitting information to the brain.

Whenever someone is experiencing fear and high stress levels, the body is primed to run away or to take a defensive stand. This is the well known fight or flight reaction. In recent years 'freeze' has been added, so we now have fight, flight or freeze. Living through a viral pandemic is stressful in many ways, but we can't run away from a virus and that leaves fight or freeze. To freeze at the sight of a snake is a good thing and could prevent being bitten. However, if coronavirus news, statistics, restrictions and uncertainties cause a person to freeze emotionally or mentally, then feelings of anxiety or fear or anger can be prolonged indefinitely. The nose 'talks' to the limbic system, so an essential oil – that is a known antidepressant or relaxant – will signal to the brain that the 'danger is over' and that there is no longer a need to be on the alert. That it is safe to relax. To let go of fear and anger, and to feel less anxious.

The fight response is an available option by choosing to be proactive. All that is necessary is to reach for an antiviral essential oil and use it. We are breathing in and out around 20,000 – 22,000 times a day, so we could use a few of those breaths to inhale antiviral essential oil vapours. I have listed twenty-one affordable and easily obtainable essential oils, each one proven to be antiviral. And because essential oils are multi-functional and multi-therapeutic, one essential oil from my list could be both antidepressant and antiviral. Many of the antiviral essential oils listed in PART 2 are well-known relaxants and antidepressants. But there is no need to 'take my word for it', just obtain a few essential oils, try one of my suggestions, and see for yourself.

Essential oils are aromatic molecules that when inhaled, travel through the nasal passages to the limbic system where the brain can identify which aroma is being inhaled. The limbic system is situated close to the olfactory epithelium cells – and as the route of infection is via the nostrils, we could be helping ourselves fight airborne pathogens by vaporising antiviral essential oils into the air – inside our homes and offices. Epithelial cells also line the trachea and lungs so that any respiratory virus, if not killed off in the nasal passages, will multiply and move down the throat, causing a cough. A cough is the body's way of attempting to expel an invading pathogen. If not killed off in the throat, a virus will keep spreading downwards until it reaches the lungs, where the disease becomes more severe. To me, it makes sense to halt any virus in its tracks.

Inhalation of antiviral essential oils can work in three distinct ways. Firstly, essential oils can change a person's mood; inhaling essential oils with proven anti-depressant properties – such as clary sage or ylang-ylang – can help a depressed person to feel better. Several essential oils – some like rosemary or lemongrass are 'energisers' and can 'perk up' the emotions. These two essential oils are very inexpensive and uplifting, but are too strong to be applied to the skin, except after mixing with a larger quantity of any carrier oil. But, for inhalation it is not necessary to dilute essential oils. Simply put a few drops of rosemary or lemongrass onto a disposable cotton pad or tissue, and hold under the nose but without the skin coming into contact with the essential oil. Inhale for a few minutes. Another time, do the same with lemongrass oil – and judge the difference in how you feel, and which of the two aromas you prefer.

Secondly, inhaling essential oils is a direct route for antiviral vapours to reach the epithelial cells of the upper nasal passages; influenza and the common cold have been successfully treated in this way – with a selection of essential oils, such as eucalyptus oil – for hundreds of years. And also, inhaling essential oils may help someone with anosmia, whether partial or complete loss of smell and taste, to regain their sense of smell. Anosmia is a common symptom of Covid-19, affecting many people, most of whom will recover their sense of smell within days or weeks; however, for some people, having recovered from an acute infection accompanied by loss of smell, this condition becomes chronic, and with no medical cure has come to be known as a common symptom of long Covid.

The antiviral essential oils
University researchers have referenced more than thirty essential oils as 'antiviral', and below I list twenty-one of them, all of which fall into the following categories: Inexpensive and commonly available from high street stores, online essential oil aromatherapy stores, and safe to use at home.

I have included one exception – lemon balm/melissa – because although it is a costly essential oil, it works very quickly to halt the progression of herpes simplex of the lips, and has a very pleasant aroma. Melissa* can be obtained as a 5% or 10% dilution in jojoba or other base oil/wax, but the 100% essential oil of melissa is very expensive due to the yield from plant material being very low compared to lavender. It takes more than seven tonnes – that's a massive 7,000 kilos of plant material to produce just one kilo of melissa oil.

Common Name	Latin Name
aniseed	pimpinella anisum
bergamot	citrus bergamia
clary sage	salvia sclarea
cinnamon	cinnamomum zeylanicum
clove	eugenia aromatica
dill	anethum graveolens
eucalyptus	eucalyptus globulus
geranium	pelargonium graveolens
ginger	zingiber officianale
juniper	juniperus communis

Common Name	Latin Name
lavender	lavandula angustifolia
lemon	citrus limonum
lemongrass	cymbopogon citratus
manuka	leptospermum scoparium
Spanish marjoram	thymus mastichina
sweet marjoram	origanum majorana
*melissa	melissa officianalis
peppermint	mentha piperita
rosemary	rosemarinus officinalis
tea tree	melaleuca alternifolia
thyme	thymus vulgaris/ thymus zygis
ylang-ylang	*cananga odorata*

Although ylang-ylang has not yet been proven antiviral, I include it here as it one of the best essential oils to treat the symptoms of depression.

On the following page, you will see the criteria I used for including or excluding antiviral essential oils.

Commonly available

Essential oils produced in large quantities and easy to find in health food shops, internet sites and aromatherapy essential oil suppliers. Rare or challenging to obtain essential oils are excluded, as are the expensive oils – with one exception – melissa as it has a delightful aroma and is perfect for treating a cold sore.

Safe to use

I have excluded essential oils that are highly irritant to the skin or mucous membranes. Also excluded are the essential oils known to be toxic, which should never be used, even by a therapist.

Non-confusing

A few essential oils are subject to dispute regarding their correct name – common or Latin – and these are also excluded.

Aroma chemicals are not part of this book, even though many are proven to be antiviral. These single chemicals taken from essential oils are not available to the general public. Essential oils – rosemary, tea tree and lavender for example – are composed of dozens of aroma chemicals – 1,8-cineole in rosemary, terpinen-4-ol in tea tree, linalool in lavender – each one is a major chemical of these three common essential oils.

Many Ayurvedic and Chinese traditional medicinal herbs are proven to be antiviral and the subject of several research papers. My book is entirely focused on essential oils.

My 'go to' essential oils/aromatherapy reference book has to be *Encyclopaedia of Essential Oils* by Julia Lawless.The book details a large selection of essential oils in an easy to navigate manner. I have the 1992 edition but a more recent version is available online.

Antiviral essential oil use
The following lists of antiviral essential oils are included for guidance only, as everyone has different preferences and tolerances. If any skin irritation or sneezing occurs with a particular essential oil, stop using it and try a different essential oil when you feel ready. Children are generally more sensitive to essential oils than adults, so always use them with caution. Specialist aromatherapy books for babies and children can be found in bookstores and online.

Vaporize into a room

aniseed, bergamot, clary sage, cinnamon leaf (not bark), clove, dill, eucalyptus, geranium, ginger, juniper, lavender, lemon, lemongrass, manuka, Spanish marjoram, sweet marjoram, peppermint, rosemary, tea tree, thyme (information on vaporising essential oils can be found on page 59).

Personal inhalation

bergamot, clary sage*, dill, eucalyptus, geranium, ginger, juniper, lemon, lavender, manuka, rosemary, tea tree (*not to be confused with common sage, which is toxic and should not be used at home).

Safe to use on the skin for massage

dill, eucalyptus, geranium, lavender, manuka, clary sage, bergamot. Bergamot is phototoxic, causing pigmentation of the skin, so avoid sunbathing after a massage.

Can cause dermal irritation on sensitive skin

aniseed, cinnamon leaf, clove, ginger, lemon, lemongrass, peppermint, tea tree, thyme

Avoid during pregnancy

aniseed, dill, juniper, rosemary, sweet marjoram, thyme,
Spanish marjoram

Suitable for 5% application to the soles of the feet

Eucalyptus, lavender, tea tree, thyme, manuka
Roller bottles are available in 2mls, 5mls and 10mls.

Irritant to mucous membranes and not recommended for baths or personal inhalation

cinnamon, clove bud, lemongrass, Spanish marjoram,
sweet marjoram, peppermint, thyme

Oils for specific uses

Depression, anxiety and other complaints brought on by nervous tension

bergamot, clary sage, geranium, juniper, lavender and
ylang-ylang*

*ylang-ylang is not one of the antiviral essential oils
but successfully reduces the symptoms of depression
and many other stress-related issues.

Relaxing oils to help with sleep problems
geranium, lavender, sweet marjoram, clary sage

Energising oils to help overcome fatigue/debility
cinnamon, eucalyptus, geranium, ginger, lemongrass, thyme, peppermint & rosemary

Essential oils for using neat on a cold sore
lavender, tea tree, melissa, a.k.a. lemon balm*. Little and often is the key, using a tiny amount of your chosen essential oil.

*melissa is a costly oil as the oil yield from plant material is very low, but is included here as a potent option for treating herpes simplex sores.

Gargling to treat a sore throat
Gargling is not for everyone, especially children, who might struggle **not** to swallow or inhale the liquid, so I am only writing this section for people who are able and willing to gargle.

My antiviral gargle consists of two drops of essential oil in water: one drop of clove and one drop of thyme added to a small glass jar, half-full of water. The jar needs to be shaken rapidly for several seconds for the essential oils to be dispersed throughout the water. Take a sip and gargle. When gargling is carried out on a regular basis – daily or a few times a week – the aromatic water reaches the back of the throat where sore throats originate and is very effective. I have experienced my sore throat getting better after just one gargle.

The choice of essential oil is yours, but any one (or two) oils from the twenty-one antiviral essential oils list will be helpful. In case of accidental swallowing of the aromatic water whilst gargling, I recommend using essential oils classified as food and drink flavourings. Lavender is a beautiful fragrance on the skin – but once, I accidentally used lavender for a gargle and found the taste to be disgusting. A small lidded jar is ideal, as the aromatic water – if used once a day – will be used up within a week or so, but if not all used, it is best to throw away the leftover and make a fresh batch. If you were not a big fan of your first choice of essential oil/s, just make another aromatic water the next time you want to gargle. Making an aromatic water 'to taste' is inexpensive. Just remember to always shake the jar vigorously before each use. And keep out of reach of children.

Nasal protection

As we all know, viruses enter the body via the nasal passages, which makes the nostrils a very important part of our defence system. Wearing a mask is important when in a public place, and I always wear mine, but on reaching home, I don't wear a mask. I don't go out very much, but my son does, and it is always possible that he could bring the virus into the house. What I do for myself and highly recommend is to coat the inside of the nostrils with an aromatic layer of protection – once a day. By aromatic layer, I mean a blend of antiviral essential oils in jojoba oil. Jojoba is a liquid wax that does not oxidise like fatty oils; it is odourless and a perfect base for essential oil blends, as they will remain in excellent condition for a long time. Some essential oils are irritant to the mucous membranes, and these should always be avoided, but any of the oils listed under the heading Personal Inhalation would be excellent. I recommend making a 1% blend of essential oil in jojoba oil. A clean fingertip is the easiest way to apply nasal protection, but as that may not be convenient for some people, a cotton bud or wedge of cotton wool with a drop or two of the aromatic liquid would also work well.

It is more convenient for me to make up a 30ml amber bottle of essential oil in jojoba mix than to make a smaller amount, simply because I am generally too busy to 'look after myself' on a daily basis. I know that jojoba and essential oils are a perfect mix, and when stored in a well-capped bottle, out of direct sunlight, can be trusted for several months, at the very least.

We don't all have access to Pyrex beakers to measure the quantity of jojoba or fatty oils, so an easy way to calculate a 1% dilution is to remember that:

One teaspoon of jojoba or carrier oil equates to 5mls.

1 or 2 drops of essential oil, added to 5mls jojoba or carrier oil, equates to a 1% dilution.

As essential oils vary in viscosity, I can't be any more accurate. However, once you start mixing, blending and using essential oils, you will soon find out what works for you. For example, you can increase or decrease the number of drops to suit you or the person for whom you are making the blend, and there are many other occasions when an aromatic layer inside the nose might be a good idea. For help with getting to sleep at bedtime – try lavender in jojoba. For treating the symptoms of anxiety or depression – try ylang-ylang in jojoba. I would be delighted to hear from anyone who has benefited from using my suggestions, as it may help other people, and I will put all recipes into the public domain via my blogsite.

For application to insect bites and stings, spots and minor burns
lavender, tea tree*.

*A small number of users have found tea tree to cause both irritation and allergic reaction

Cold compress – to reduce a fever
eucalyptus, lavender
These two essential oils are written about in detail on pages 20 and 21.

For personal inhalation

Inhaling essential oils directly over a bowl of hot water is more intense than breathing in aromatic vapours that are diffusing into a room, so ensure that you like the aroma. Also, ensure that the essential oil does not come under the heading of 'irritant to mucous membranes.' Add one or two drops of antiviral essential oils to a mug or bowl of hot but not boiling water, lean over and take deep breaths, but if coughing occurs then stop using, and choose a new oil. Repeat once or twice a day but ensure that energising oils are not used in the evening as they could interfere with getting to sleep. Restrict your choice of essential oils to the ones you are comfortable with and know to be safe to use. If the use of essential oils in hot water does not appeal, there is the option of buying personal inhalers, online.

For vaporizing a room

Essential oils that should not be used on the skin because they are known to irritate, may be diffused into a room to lessen the volume of airborne viruses. Diffusers – mains or battery operated – can vary from a few pounds to over a hundred pounds. Yet, without spending any money, it is easy to diffuse an antiviral essential oil into a room by adding two or three drops to a mug of hot (but not boiling) water. I regard this as a simple preventative measure and a cost-effective way to help purify the immediate indoor environment – ideal for use during 'lockdown' or throughout the winter when doors and windows are closed and fresh air can't circulate indoors. A more comprehensive range of antiviral essential oils can be vaporized into a room than can be used for personal inhalation. But if a household member has a chronic respiratory ailment, suffers from epilepsy, or is hypersensitive to aromatic products, then seek advice before vaporizing any room they might be using. If necessary, wait for the household member to leave their room, as it could be preferable to vaporize an empty bedroom. Whether a mug of hot water or a diffuser is used, add your selected essential oil/s, leave the room with the door closed, and return an hour or so later to open the window for a few minutes, allowing fresh air in and residual vapours to leave. It could be the case that individual household members have their own favourite antiviral essential oil, and it would be so simple to have a bespoke, vaporized environment. If anyone in the household has asthma or other chronic respiratory condition, then the choice of essential oil may need to be restricted , so best to check with a health professional before diffusing essential oils into the home.

A vaporizer/diffuser is a good investment once you know that essential oils vapours in your home are acceptable to you and your household. I have an inexpensive diffuser with an internal container for adding water and essential oils, and yet the machine does not create dampness. The reason is that the device also contains an ultrasonic component that pulverizes the droplets of water and essential oils to create a very fine mist that is sent upwards and out into a room. I like to add 6 or 7 drops of essential oil such as clary sage or rosemary, run the machine for half an hour or so and switch off when the atmosphere in my room is pleasant. Sometimes, I use a blend of citrus oils – 2 drops of lime, 2 drops of orange and 2-3 drops of lemon. We are all individuals, so what suits one person may not be acceptable to someone else. Possibly, because I am attuned to working with essential oils, I find that leaving my diffuser running for about an hour is my maximum, after which time I have to switch it off as I begin to feel slightly nauseous. Trial and error is a good thing, and as the twenty-one antiviral essential oils listed on pages 48–49 are inexpensive to buy, finding an ideal blend or a single aroma that is much appreciated should not be a big financial gamble.

Bathing

An aromatic bath is a wonderful thing – but only if an unwell person has the strength to run a bath to the perfect temperature, dilute essential oils in a teaspoon of unscented shower gel, mix thoroughly in the water and then climb in. If I felt unwell, I would leave that pleasure until I had sufficient energy to undertake what would generally be a simple task, but post-Covid might seem like a big deal. Always choose essential oils that are non-irritant to the skin and also not an irritant to mucous membranes. For a relaxing bath, use up to six drops of essential oil, but choose those essential oils known to have calming/sedative properties and that are skin-friendly. Everyone will have a slightly different skin tolerance to essential oils in the bath, so in general, it is advisable to mix essential oil drops into a small amount of fragrance-free shower gel and disperse thoroughly in the water.

Massage

Because essential oils are concentrated, they must always be dissolved in a carrier oil, and a good selection of nut and seed oils are available from health food shops. But if the only fatty oil available is from your kitchen, then that would do. Always dilute essential oils in a carrier oil for massage of large areas such as a back massage, massage of the legs, or massage of the neck and chest. The general advice is to keep to a ratio of 1%–2% essential oil to the carrier oil.

There are a few exceptions regarding the 1%–2% rule. For example, to treat a cold sore, it is acceptable to use an undiluted essential oil such as lemon, tea tree or melissa by putting a single drop onto the side of a cotton bud (rather than the tip) and applying gently by touching the cotton bud to the blister. The sooner treatment starts, the better, as an early application of antiviral essential oil can prevent cold sores from becoming more prominent and unsightly. Dispose of the used cotton tip hygienically. Other exceptions include the use of neat lavender oil on an insect bite or sting. Lavender has also been used successfully as first aid for minor burns.

Roller bottle with 5% essential oil blend

For anyone who has difficulty in falling asleep or who wakes up in the middle of the night and can't get back to sleep again, I recommend keeping a roller bottle of lavender essential oil in a base of jojoba near the bed. Jojoba does not oxidize like fatty oils, so it never goes rancid even if infrequently used, and lavender oil is my first choice nighttime essential oil. Simply roll the gentle aroma across the soles of the feet.

I recommend jojoba because it is a liquid wax and doesn't oxidize like fatty oils. There is nothing more unappealing than to remove the lid from a massage blend and find that it smells rancid. The only thing to do with a bottle of rancid massage oil is to throw it away, and that is why I invest in jojoba oil even though it is more expensive than any of the nut and seed oils.

A 5% blend of essential oils for application to the feet is an exception to the general 1%–2% dilution rule simply because the soles of adult feet have layers of toughened skin. As many people have sensitive soles and are 'ticklish' it may be preferable to apply the 5% blend to the hands and then to firmly massage the feet.

To a roller bottle, add jojoba oil, leaving enough space for the essential oils. A 10ml bottle holds two teaspoons of jojoba. Add up to 20 drops of one essential oil or mix several different essential oils to make a total of 20 drops – geranium blends very well with lavender. You decide the strength. It is easy to make the blend a bit stronger by adding more drops of essential oil.

Aromatic waters for making a compress

Essential oils will readily dissolve/blend into fatty oil but will not dissolve in water. However, it is easy to make aromatic water, and complete details are found in PART 1.

Not for internal use

Of great importance is to understand that essential oils can cause damage to the stomach and intestinal lining if consumed, so please do not take essential oils internally.

To make simple blends

Essential oils must always be diluted in a fatty base oil before using for a massage.

A massage blend is always a mix of essential oils that are diluted in a base oil. Base oils are also known as – carrier oils, fatty oils, vegetable oils, nut oils, seed oils. A massage base could also be a non-fragranced body lotion.

One teaspoon of base oil is approximately 5mls.

Two teaspoons of base oil is approximately 10mls.

1% blend in a 10ml bottle
- Base oil such as jojoba oil (or base oil of your choice)
- 1 or 2 drops directly from essential oil bottle with integral dropper.

2% blend in a 10ml bottle
- Base oil
- 2–4 drops of essential oil.

5% blend in a 10ml bottle
- Base oil of your choice
- 5–10 drops of essential oil
- I recommend a 5% blend for application to soles of the feet only.

Most essential oils come in dark glass bottles with an integral dropper, but as dropper sizes vary, I give an approximate dosage of essential oil to the base oil. Also, I wouldn't want anyone to think that the blend is useless if an extra drop is included. So, the above is an average guide. You decide what strength suits you. Bear in mind that older people may have more sensitive skin than young people. And that a blend for a child should be roughly half the amount of essential oil as for an adult.

To treat the symptoms of long Covid

Long Covid is not a disease – it is a list of post-Covid symptoms that vary in complexity from person to person. Long Covid shares many similarities with Chronic Fatigue Syndrome (ME). Currently, there is no medical cure for long Covid, and neither is there an essential oil cure. However, treating the symptoms of a disease is what modern medicine does daily, and we can do the same for long Covid, but with essential oils instead of pharmaceutical drugs. As such, we have more choice in the way we handle the symptoms of long Covid. To seek medical advice for each symptom would perhaps necessitate a prescription for multiple drugs after many visits to consultants. Instead, you can buy a selection of essential oils and use them in versatile ways, which would provide a gentle and less expensive way of finding a road back to good health.

Age is not a factor in suffering from long Covid. Young and old alike can be affected equally. More women than men have long Covid, but common to all ages and genders, the most widely experienced symptoms include fatigue, brain fog, depression, shortness of breath, diarrhoea, visual problems, anosmia and parosmia (a distorted sense of smell). Approximately 65% of people with coronavirus will develop chronic anosmia. And 10% of those people will go on to develop parosmia – when common aromas smell awful.

Over many decades of using essential oils, I have learned which essential oils work on the body, the brain and emotions. This knowledge gives me the confidence to state that every essential oil mentioned in *Antiviral Aromatherapy* could, in one way or another, help to relieve symptoms of long Covid.

If I were suffering from long Covid, I would be using essential oils every day in one way or another. For example, if I had anosmia, I would be inhaling antiviral essential oils several times a day. As I have – for many decades – turned to preventative medicine at the first signs of ill-health, I would be massaging diluted skin-safe essential oils into my neck and upper chest area. Below are some of my suggestions for treating symptoms of long Covid, but bear in mind that long Covid is 'the new kid on the block', and no one has a voice of authority. However, many people are currently conducting trials and collating helpful information, hoping that results will help many long Covid sufferers.

Fatigue and brain fog symptoms could be relieved by the regular use of rosemary, lemongrass and thyme essential oils, as they are energizing and uplifting oils. The simplest way to utilize the oils is by adding a drop or two of your chosen oil onto a tissue. Sniff uplifting and antiviral essential oils periodically during the first half of the day. Later in the day, switch to essential oils that are still antiviral but more relaxing – such as geranium and clary sage. Eucalyptus and bergamot are two oils I would use at any time of day. I have been informed that many sufferers admit that long Covid has caused them to be incapable of following a television programme, completely losing track of what they have been watching as their mental fatigue/brain fog makes it impossible to concentrate.

Should I be in that mental state, I would keep a few essential oils next to me when watching a TV programme to experiment with a different oil each day – sniffing one essential oil a couple of times while watching a film/programme, just to see if it helped with recall. And I would make a note of which oil helped by keeping a notebook and pen alongside the essential oils.

Intestinal symptoms such as indigestion, diarrhoea, stomach ache, nausea, lack of appetite are all common symptoms of long Covid. Peppermint oil has been tried and tested for many years and would be my 'go to' essential oil, as I can't think of a better essential oil than peppermint for easing problems in the digestive system. Peppermint capsules are available online or from pharmacies, and the essential oil of peppermint can be found in health food stores or online (read instructions for ways to use). Peppermint oil is antispasmodic and can quickly calm intestinal muscles that have tensed up. It works so well that doctors have already recommended it for the treatment of Irritable Bowel Syndrome. IBS is caused by cramping of the intestines or because of an overly sensitive gut. Stress is a major causative factor.

Depression often goes hand in hand with fatigue because the brain is every bit as overtired as the body. Essential oils, known to have anti-depressant properties, could help lift a heavy feeling – but gently and simply. Choosing an essential oil known to help relieve depression – such as ylang-ylang oil that has not been proven antiviral – would always be my first choice and is so easy to use. Simply put a drop onto the palm of one hand, rub the hands together, then cup the hands over the nose and mouth, and breathe in. I would inhale ylang-ylang aromas for several minutes at a time. Or drip a few drops of the oil onto a tissue and inhale the uplifting aroma. Another way of inhaling ylang-ylang (or any essential oil of your choice) is by adding a few drops of oil to a diffuser to scent the living space. But like any essential oil, if used too often over a long period, the body will tell you to stop by causing a cough or making you feel a little nauseous. Used respectfully, this is a very safe and inexpensive way of relieving symptoms of depression. Clary sage is another excellent essential oil for the relief of depression.

Anxiety is a form of fear, and fear often causes tension in the body. It will differ from person to person, but for me, the area I would always work on first is the solar plexus – where my tension seems to be stored. The place to massage is just below the rib cage and just above the navel, conveniently placed for self-massage – with diluted essential oils in a carrier base oil, A circular massage movement, with the fingertips, is the best way to begin, as stored tension can be painful and the solar plexus very sensitive. After a few minutes, I like to place both hands across my torso with elbows out to the sides – so that the fingertips of both hands are facing each other – and then apply gentle fingertip pressure into the solar plexus as you breathe out – and hold for a few seconds. Too much pressure will be uncomfortable, so only use enough for your comfort level. This is the easiest way for me to reduce tension in my body whenever life throws up stressful challenges. Relaxing oils such as lavender, geranium, clary sage, or bergamot would be my choice.

Anosmia – the medical word for loss of smell – is a common side effect of Covid-19 infection. It might be a wrong guess, but I would assume that some viral particles were still in the nasal passages if that was my situation. So, I would be applying a very dilute antiviral essential oil blend inside the nostrils. I would do this at least twice a day, once in the morning and again before going to bed for the night, and hope that my actions were going to be helpful in my process of recovery. To avoid itching/irritation use essential oils that are known to be safe on the mucous membranes.

Sleep difficulties – being unable to drop off to sleep or waking up after a few short hours and not going back to sleep is not fun. But, I have always resisted the temptation to buy OTC sleep remedies, preferring to trust the essential oils known to be relaxing. Lavender, geranium and clary sage come into this category and are also antiviral. So, I would make a 5% blend of these essential oils, either a single oil or a mix of two or three oils in jojoba. Pour the blended oils into a roller bottle and apply to the soles of the feet just before going to bed. I keep a pair of loose cotton socks to wear whenever using oils on my feet

– to prevent oil from soiling bed linen and to minimise natural dispersal of the essential oil.

Visual problems such as blurred vision or even hallucinations have joined the growing list of long Covid symptoms. In this instance, I would make up a simple massage blend – a 1% dilution of essential oils in jojoba oil – and massage thoroughly but gently into the back of my neck and hairline, behind the ears, and then I would massage my temples. On another day, I would rub the oil blend into my forehead, especially the sinus points just above the eyebrows and at the side of the nose and across to the cheekbones. My choice of essential oils would be lavender, geranium and bergamot, as I would suspect inflammation in my head or neck. I would want to choose essential oils that were both physically and emotionally soothing. Another time I would massage the oil blend into the nape of my neck, and see what works. There are some extremely severe symptoms associated with long Covid, and anyone suffering from unusual or concerning symptoms should always consult a medical professional before using essential oils.

PART 3
THE IMMUNE SYSTEM – AND WHY IT MATTERS

In the first two parts of this book, I have written about antiviral essential oils and how they work alongside the immune system to effectively fight infection.

This section will focus on the immune system and lymphatic system – body functions that work together to protect humans from pathogens such as viruses and bacteria. Knowledge of the virus that has created a catastrophic pandemic is now a part of our everyday lives through the mediums of television, newspapers, and tech gadgetry. Newsfeeds provide us with a comprehensive understanding of what the coronavirus looks like, how it works, how it can make some people very sick very quickly, and how it can take lives in a matter of days. But, although there is much talk about the importance of a vaccine to confer protection by stimulating an immune response, there seems to be very little information on the function of the immune system: how it works, what damages it and what we can do to respect and work with our 'protector'. If we can unwittingly damage the immune system, we can consciously make efforts to repair it so that it will protect us. I say this in a general manner, but I must point out that there are people – such as transplant recipients – who don't have a functioning immune system as, of necessity, they need to receive life-saving immunosuppressant drugs.

What is the immune system?

Vital though it is, many people lack an understanding of the workings of the immune system. My opinion is that we seem to know more about the solar system than we do about the immune system, so, long-winded though this section may seem, the information I have gathered explains a very complex bodily function that we can't see or feel, but without which human beings would not exist today. Long ago wiped out by viruses and bacteria. The subject of the immune system should be taught in schools as part of secondary education, as knowledge of how to stay healthy and alive seems to me, far more important than many of the mandatory facts and figures that children are required to learn, such as algebra. I can't think of anything more important than understanding the role that the immune system plays in keeping human beings alive, what damages it and what strengthens it, and why having respect for it could be the key to a long and healthy life.

The three parts of the whole

The body's ability to fight infection comprises three different systems, each working together to create the immune system. There is the lymphatic system, the innate immune system, and the acquired/adaptive immune system. I will use the 'acquired' rather than 'adaptive' throughout this book to avoid confusion. Acquired immunity comes from having and surviving an illness. The body remembers what that illness looked like so that the next time the disease attacks the body, the immune system works fast to eliminate the infection and prevent the person from getting sick.

Vaccination has a similar effect in priming the body to fight a particular virus. At the time of writing this book, it is the 2019 coronavirus that the acquired immune system is learning to protect us from by producing antibodies (chemicals) that detect and kill particular foreign invaders – as the body is SELF, and all invading organisms are NON-SELF.

The innate immune system is what we have had from birth – immune cells from the mother's birth canal and then colostrum, the pre-milk liquid that babies can suckle as soon as they are born – which confers some immunity as we are growing up. In 1918, my mother was a seven-year-old who survived an infection of influenza when many millions of people around the world were dying from the Spanish flu. As it was a strain of influenza that had never been encountered before, it quickly caused a global pandemic. My mother's eldest sister – my aunt Mary – nursed her parents and siblings back to full health before succumbing to influenza herself. Exhausted from nursing her family members day and night over many days, she became ill with the flu and died at the age of twenty-one. Her immune system had become severely depleted and no longer capable of fighting off the virus.

My mother was at primary school when she caught the Spanish flu, and she remained free of influenza for the rest of her life, passing away at the age of 95. In her late 80s, her doctors insisted on administering an annual flu vaccine. Yet, prior to that medical intervention, she had managed to avoid catching the flu for seven decades without a vaccine. I now have an understanding of the wonders of the immune system, but as a child, I was always mystified that I, along with my brother and sister, would all 'go down with the flu' from time to time – but our mother never became infected with influenza.

Now for the hard facts
Although there are some differences, the lymphatic system is a part of the immune system (innate and acquired). The individual systems work together to create a single system that is constantly monitoring the body. I think of it in terms of a railway analogy. The lymphatic system can be described as a kind of railway network, with interconnecting rails, sleepers, stations, signals, engineers, and personnel to organise the running and repair of the entire network.

The immune system is like the trains that travel on the railway network; everything needed to transport people and goods – the engines and carriages, the interior seats and toilets and spaces for bicycles, wheelchairs, and buggies. Then the personnel to operate the trains – drivers, guards, ticket inspectors, porters, refreshment cart employees, and all the engineers needed to repair and upgrade the tracks and trains, cleaners, provision of electricity... the list goes on. Neither one system would be of any use without the other. They need to form a cohesive service to facilitate a vital function.

The lymphatic/immune system has developed over many thousands of years to provide human beings with one vital function – that of identifying, attacking, and destroying any threats to the health of the human. This involves transporting B cells, T cells, NK cells, and much more around the body to attack and destroy invading viruses, bacteria, and other pathogens. The body's own cells are not attacked as they are recognised as SELF, but the immune system sees anything identified as NON-SELF as a target to be destroyed. As well as invading pathogens, many types of cancer cells are also destroyed. Humans would die very quickly if the immune system stopped working entirely. For example, when my eldest daughter was undergoing chemotherapy, the drugs caused neutropenia – the death of neutrophils – more details under Cancer sub-heading, page 89 – that coincided with with her two children coming down with chickenpox. She was told emphatically by her doctor to "get the children out of the house; their infection could kill you."

For ease of understanding, I have provided a simplified outline of this rather complicated process below.

- The purpose of the immune system is to identify and protect the body SELF from foreign particles NON-SELF that are not produced by the body.

- When the immune system detects NON-SELF it produces antigens.

- The immune system is comprised of the innate and acquired immune systems and the lymphatic system. Although fulfilling separate functions, they intrinsically work in harmony with each other.

- The lymphatic vessels begin as capillaries, which feed into larger lymphatic vessels that ultimately empty into the bloodstream via a series of ducts.

- That journey takes lymph through nodes dotted throughout the body but which are primarily found in the groin, armpits, neck, chest, and abdomen.

- Humans have about 500–600 lymph nodes throughout the body.

- Lymph is not actively pumped by the heart but forced through vessels by means of bodily movements, such as muscle contractions and breathing.

- A system of one-way valves keeps lymph moving towards the heart.

- Lymph merges with the circulatory system via lymph ducts in the neck.

- Lymph nodes are bean-shaped tissues dotted along the lymphatic pipes where they act as filters, trapping viruses and other germs.

- Swollen lymph nodes indicate that the immune system is actively working to fight infection.

- The skin and mucous membranes, areas of the body exposed to the world, form the first line of defence against viral invasion.

- The innate immune response is powered by a lymphocyte known as a natural killer cell.

- A natural killer (NK) cell circulates through the bloodstream, and its cytotoxic (cell-killing) properties work in combination with T cells.

- NK cells are one of the body's first-line defences against viruses.

- NK cells do not kill viruses and other pathogens but attack and destroy human cells that are infected with viruses.

- The innate immune system is more ancient than the acquired immune system.

- When the innate immune system notices a new pathogen, it activates the acquired immune system by sending a chemical message.

- The innate immune system works faster than the acquired: minutes to hours for the innate system, but days to weeks for the acquired.

- Innate immunity is composed of the skin, enzymes, epithelial membranes, mucous membranes, NK cells, plus most of the white blood cells – in particular neutrophils that are first responders to the site of a new infection.

- One hundred billion neutrophils are produced in the bone marrow every day.

- Dendritic cells form a bridge between the innate and the acquired immune systems, allowing a comprehensive flow of immunity.

- The acquired immune response involves many cell types but is primarily controlled by lymphocytes, one of the many white blood cells that are collectively called leucocytes.

- The human body contains approximately 1,000,000,000,000 (or one trillion) lymphocytes.

- B cells produce antibodies. Antibodies patrol through the lymphatic system ready to destroy pathogens that are recognised as a danger to health.

- T cells communicate with other cells of the acquired immune system, with instructions to destroy cells infected with viruses (or other pathogens).

- Both B cells and T cells develop from bone marrow. B cells mature in the bone marrow while T cells migrate from the bone marrow to the thymus gland where they mature.

- Both types of cells are constantly circulating throughout the bloodstream and lymph, passing through lymph nodes, creating a highly effective defence against invaders.

- The thymus resides above the heart and behind the breastbone. T cells constantly travel around the body, monitoring the surfaces of all cells looking for changes.

- Other parts of the immune system include the spleen, the epithelial cells of the respiratory tract, the tonsils and most importantly, the mucous membranes – because, although we can live without our tonsils or spleen – we could not live without the mucous membranes of the bowel, where more than half of the body's antibodies can be found.

- The large bowel contains harmless bacteria, known as gut flora, or more recently being referred to as 'the biome'. (More about the biome later).

- Damage to the immune system prevents it from keeping track of viruses and other pathogens, including cancer cells. Humans could not live without an immune system, and because of its importance, it makes sense to understand it, have respect for it, and know what damages it.

What damages the immune system?

Fundamentally, the immune system only repairs itself when we are asleep, and therefore, the primary damage to a person's immune system comes from not getting enough sleep, or getting poor quality or disturbed sleep. Other factors that impair the immune system include:

- Stressful life situations, such as lack of adequate finances, lack of support, overworking, living in an unhealthy environment, loneliness ... and numerous other worrying personal situations that could fill the pages of this book.

- Constant worry about the state of world health, the economy, wars, climate change and a desire for peace that seems unobtainable.

- Grief is a major stressor to the body. Whenever someone dear to us dies, the body struggles to process the loss, using up a considerable amount of energy and significantly disrupting the ability to sleep.

- Nurses and doctors become ill whenever their immune system is under-performing due to stressful working conditions, overworking and a lack of sleep. But sadly, this comes with the job. We, collectively, as taxpayers and intelligent human beings, should find this unacceptable. Even in a war zone, military personnel are given 'r&r' time. Rest and recuperation are recognised as a necessity for health and good performance – both mental and physical. Yet hospital doctors and nurses work a rota system – which in itself is stressful for the body to cope with. With variable working hours and variable sleeping hours, their bodies can't get into a rhythm. And the working of the body is all about rhythms – in particular, I am thinking about the production of melatonin that is responsible for allowing human beings to fall asleep

- **Immunosuppressants.** Anyone who has been the recipient of an organ transplant will require immunosuppressants. This necessary intervention prevents the immune system from doing its job – which is recognising the transplant as NON-SELF and attacking it. Persons with an autoimmune disease also need to take immunosuppressants.

- **Cancer.** Patients undergoing chemotherapy always have a depleted immune system, as most chemotherapy drugs are designed to destroy fast-growing cells. Cancer cells grow rapidly, but so do neutrophils. Neutrophils, produced in the bone marrow at a rate of 100 billion every day, are obliterated by cancer drugs, resulting in a condition known as neutropenia. A severely damaged immune system is the outcome.

- **Antibiotics.** They are your enemy unless you are infected with very powerful bacteria – for example, strep throat, meningitis, gangrene. So, antibiotics should only be taken when absolutely necessary. Avoid whenever possible, as it can take up to two years for the biome to be fully repaired. The microbiome is an integral part of the immune system. Not only are antibiotics damaging to the immune system but inappropriate usage is seen as a major cause of drug-resistant infections. Repairs to the immune system can only take place when we sleep.

All of the above can damage the immune system, but it can be repaired over a period of time. The most important thing to remember is that above all else, there is a fundamental necessity for good sleep – eight hours sleep in a dark room is the ideal, as the immune system is only capable of carrying out repairs whilst we are asleep. I think of it as the London Underground. When I travelled on the London Underground daily for work, I experienced the crowded carriages, the newspapers and the ceiling straps to hold onto when no seats were vacant. What I didn't experience but took for granted were all of the tasks such as cleaning, repairs and inspection of tunnels and platforms. Jobs that can only take place during the night, when stations are locked and trains are stationary.

The difference between viruses and bacteria

Does the immune system discriminate between viruses and bacteria? The short answer is 'no'. But there is a difference in numbers, and this, in general, is the difference between the immune system's ability to protect the human host – or not.

There is a vast difference. Generally speaking, bacteria increase in number by dividing themselves in two. So, assuming they double in number every 24 hours, bacteria multiply as follows:

Monday	There is only one
Tuesday	Two
Wednesday	Four
Thursday	Eight
Friday	Sixteen
Saturday	Thirty-two
Sunday	Sixty-four

It is easy to see that bacterial growth is relatively slow. Although some, such as intestinal bacteria, can quickly become life-threatening, there is generally a measured pace to a bacterial infection.

Viruses, on the other hand, have a fast growth rate. Viral multiplication is very different from bacterial, as a virus does not divide itself. To multiply, a virus needs to invade a human cell (HOST). It reproduces itself inside the human cell and then breaks out. I am going to be very simple with my calculations and assume that every virus, once inside a human cell, creates 100 copies of itself. And I will assume that this process takes 24 hours. In the case of coronavirus, what I know to be a scientific fact is that replication only takes place inside the epithelial cells of the respiratory system. My calculations are simplistic and serve only as an example for comparing bacterial growth versus viral replication.

Monday. One virus invades one human cell (HOST), where it replicates itself by 100.

Tuesday. The host cell bursts open, releasing 100 viruses. Each invades a host cell.

Wednesday. One hundred host cells x 100 viruses per cell burst open, releasing 10,000 viruses.

Thursday. 10,000 viruses invade 10,000 human cells, creating 10,000 x 100 = 1,000,000 viruses.

Friday. One million viruses enter a further one million host cells where they replicate x 100 creating one hundred million viruses.

Saturday. One hundred million viruses invade one hundred million host cells; each cell multiplies by 100. Bursting out comes ten billion viruses.

Sunday. There will be one trillion viruses. Monday, there will be one hundred trillion. From then on my calculator can't cope!

Conclusion

Awareness of the speed at which the coronavirus multiplies demonstrates how vulnerable human beings are to quickly becoming overwhelmed by a new virus. And that is why I have written this book; to let people know that we could and should be looking to Mother

Nature for help. Essential oils, the backbone of aromatherapy, are powerful aromatic tools that enable us to work in harmony with the immune system to fight infection.

Mother Nature's Pharmacy is available to all of us – but must be used respectfully and safely. PART 2 of this book gives all the details necessary to use essential oils. There is ample information to use potent plant antivirals confidently within the home in order to combat airborne viral particles while self-isolating. And in general, to be proactive against the virus in an effort to stay free of infection. There are various ways that essential oils, when diluted, can be used on specific body parts at the first sign of swollen glands, a cough, or a sore throat. To be proactive makes more sense than sitting and hoping. Knowledge of which essential oils work, in what dilution and in which particular way could be an asset for you and your family.

PART 4
INTERNATIONAL SCIENTIFIC RESEARCH

This part of my book looks at the mounting evidence of essential oils as potential antivirals. It refers to individual university trials conducted to determine which of the many essential oils in the world are antiviral. When an essential oil is found – through rigorous testing procedures – to be antiviral, it is then usual for further research to take place in order to find out how it works. Is it the vapour that is potent? Or is it the liquid oil that is responsible? Sometimes, research takes place with the individual constituents that make up an essential oil. This research determines whether one of the individual constituents has more significant antiviral activity than the whole essential oil. When referring to a potent essential oil in many aromatherapy books, the general expression is "the whole is greater than the sum of its parts". The opposite could be true in virology. Several in silico research papers find that major constituents of essential oil, such as linalool – found in several different essential oils – should undergo further research. The challenge for Big Pharma is to develop a drug that kills a virus but that doesn't do too much damage to the host. That's you and me.

In the following pages, I refer to published, available university research – whether in vitro or in silico – by the **country** in which the research took place. Reading through dozens of research papers and finding references to the many previously published trials with essential oils, could have resulted in me writing a 'text book', but my intention has always been to keep the book small and simple with information clear and on-point. However, to enable further reading for anyone interested in the different approaches employed by scientists to provide irrefutable evidence of the antiviral efficacy of essential oils. I have given full references in the Citations section that follows PART 4. I am delighted to see that antiviral essential oil research has become international, mirroring the current viral pandemic. I sincerely hope that each member of every research team gets the respect and accolade they deserve for their diligent work and forward thinking. And for anyone wishing to find an answer to the million-dollar question of "how do essential oils breach the outer defences of viruses?" information on the subject of membrane disruption research follows the **country** research.

Before I write about antiviral research from individual universities, I want to explain some of the terminology involved for anyone like me who is non-scientifically trained. There are three main types of microbiology research.

Introduction to scientific terminology

1. in vitro – is research in laboratory glassware, such as a Petri dish that Julius Petri invented in the late 1800s. The common form of microbiology testing.

2. in vivo – is research with animals. Generally, the testing is done with mice.

3. in silico – is research utilising computer modelling: analysing prior published in vitro papers with proven antiviral evidence for a

select number of essential oils, and then hypothesising a potential use for these oils in the treatment of SARS-CoV-2 – but only after further in vitro research has taken place with the coronavirus and antiviral essential oils.

Virology is a specialist branch of microbiology. Most universities have microbiology labs, but bacteria and viruses cannot be worked on in the same laboratory. Virology research is less common.

- A virus can be DNA or RNA.

- A virus can be enveloped or non-enveloped.

- Enveloped viruses are encased in a lipid membrane.

- Non-enveloped viruses are enclosed in protein.

- The herpes simplex virus is DNA.

- The influenza virus is RNA.

- Coronaviruses are RNA.

- In a few of the university papers the terms, GLC and MS are used.

- GLC is Gas-Liquid Chromatography – it identifies the individual aroma chemicals of essential oils.

- MS is Mass Spectrometry – and determines the quantity of each individual aromatic chemical.

- *Virion can mean the whole virus or viral particle/ cytotoxicity means damage caused to human cells/in microbiology research papers essential oils are often referred to as drugs.*

Coronaviruses and rhinoviruses are responsible for the common cold, and were first identified in the 1960s, but considered mild as none had caused any severe infection. The 2019 coronavirus was new, which meant that no one had any immunity to it, and for that reason, vaccines were quickly developed and authorised by government health bodies.

Essential oils don't seem to discriminate between DNA and RNA viruses.

The individual constituents that compose an essential oil are known by many names – aroma chemicals – aroma compounds – constituent parts – aromatic compounds – chemical constituents – component parts. But they all mean the same thing – the individual aromatic chemicals that make up an essential oil.

More than two dozen university research papers have been referenced from the many published articles to be found online. And from a very long list of essential oils (and their individual constituents) proven to be antiviral, I have listed only the readily available essential oils, low cost and safe to use at home. See details in PART 2. Aroma chemicals are not part of this book as these single chemicals taken from essential oils do not meet the above criteria.

Historically, pharmaceutical products were derived from botanical plants and today, botanical preparations still account for the basis of at least 25% of the pharmaceutical products sold in pharmacies and used by hospitals and clinics. These days, pharmaceutical companies generally work with a single active chemical (natural or synthetic) or a well-defined mixture of chemicals, but can only invest time and money if a patent is granted. Of critical importance in a patent filing process is to demonstrate 'novel use', and for that reason, traditionally used aromatic plants and essential oils are of little interest, as Mother Nature cannot be patented. So, while we are waiting for Big Pharma to create and market medicine for the prevention or cure of Covid-19, we can be utilising antiviral essential oils in our daily lives – for our health and wellbeing. The following pages will, I hope, act as a snapshot of the available scientific activity with essential oils versus common viruses. As you read through PART 4 it is not necessary to understand the science as each antiviral essential oil is in bold, and this is what I want to show you.

Antiviral in vitro research

Canada, 2014. Researchers in Vancouver set up laboratory trials to evaluate the possible antiviral activity of essential oils and essential oil vapours against the influenza virus. 'Influenza viruses continue to pose threats of epidemics, resulting from mutated viruses to which we have inadequate remedies... alternative therapies that target the actual virus rather than a specific gene might be more useful.' Some previously published research papers 'had demonstrated effective ...antiviral properties in experimental conditions, but most of the studies only tested the liquid oil phase.' As the vapour phase of essential oils had not been tested, this trial tested nine essential oils – in the vapour phase – along with major components of the essential oils.

A liquid phase is when the liquid essential oil is trialled against pathogens. The vapour phase (sometimes called the 'gaseous phase') is when an essential oil is dispersed into a glass cabinet containing airborne viruses.

The research team evaluated several essential oils and some of the major constituents for their potential anti-influenza virus properties in both liquid and vapour phase. The research looked at antiviral effects of vapour on the influenza virus after 10 minutes and 30 minutes, and in the vapour phase showed no adverse effects on human epithelial cells. Cinnamon, however, should not be used on the skin, as even in dilution, it is a well-known skin irritant.

Bergamot. Cinnamon. Eucalyptus. Geranium. Lavender. Lemongrass. Thyme. Seven of the nine essential oils tested were proven to be antiviral. The two non-antiviral oils were cypress and sage. All Essential oils tested are commonly available. The fastest-acting essential oils were **cinnamon leaf***, **bergamot**, **common thyme**, and **lemongrass** in the liquid phase. In the published paper, the researchers refer to these essential oils as virucidal – indicating an ability to kill the virus rather than merely inhibiting its growth. Also of note is the evidence that **cinnamon**, **bergamot** and **lemongrass** displayed 100% inhibition of the virus yet did not damage human epithelial cells (in trials); however, some essential oils can irritate mucous membranes.

Bergamot and **eucalyptus** were active against the influenza virus after 10 minutes of exposure in the vapour phase. **Geranium, cinnamon*** and **lemongrass** were active within 30 minutes of exposure. **Lavender, eucalyptus** and **geranium** reduced the viral load by at least 80%.

*Cinnamon oils (leaf and bark) are too strong for use on the skin. Cinnamon essential oils are irritant to the skin and should be avoided in massage blends even though they are widely used in small amounts in the food and drinks industry.

Overall results with essential oils and the influenza H1N1 virus proved the research objective: essential oil vapours could be effective antivirals even with essential oils that are known irritants to the skin.

Germany, 2001. The research team examined the antiviral effect of two Australian essential oils – **tea tree** and **eucalyptus** – against herpes simplex viruses. Assessment of toxicity to human cells proved to be moderate. The in vitro testing was by plaque assay reduction, which means 'each infectious virus particle multiplies under conditions that result in a localised area of infected cells...revealed as areas of destroyed cells.' '**Tea tree** exhibited high levels of virucidal activity against both HSV-1 and 2, with plaque reduction at 93.0% to 98.2%.' **Eucalyptus** oil exhibited distinct but less antiviral activity than **tea tree** oil in another trial, but overall results indicate that '**tea tree** and **eucalyptus**

oils affect the virus before or during adsorption, but not after penetration into the host cell'. Concluding 'although the active anti-herpes components of **tea tree** and **eucalyptus** oils are not yet known, their possible application as antiviral agents in recurrent herpes infection is promising.'

Germany, 2003. Peppermint essential oil was the subject of examination against herpes simplex types 1 and 2 through a plaque reduction assay. '**Peppermint** oil exhibited high levels of virucidal activity – against both types – in viral suspension tests.' And in another test, plaque formation was significantly reduced by 82%–92%. A time-dependent trial demonstrated 99% antiviral activity. Overall results indicate that **peppermint** oil affected the virus before penetration into a human cell but not afterwards. In conclusion, the researchers state, 'considering the lipophilic nature of the oil which allows it to penetrate the skin, **peppermint** oil might be suitable for topical therapeutic use as a virucidal agent in recurrent herpes infection.'

Germany, 2005. In this research paper with the herpes simplex virus, the oil under review was **manuka**

essential oil and its two main aromatic compounds. Initial tests were with the whole essential oil and assessments made at varying times during the infection cycle. Both types of the virus (HSV-1 and HSV-2) were found to be inhibited by manuka. Results varied but 'both HSV types were significantly inhibited when the viruses were pre-treated with manuka oil... before cell infection.' 'At non-toxic (to human cells) levels, **manuka** was effective against plaque formation in both types of virus, significantly reducing type 1 by 99.5% and type 2 by 98.9 %.' 'After virus penetration into the host cells, replication of HSV-1 particle was inhibited to about 41% by **manuka** oil.' Tests with the two main constituents of **manuka** 'inhibited the virulence of HSV-1 in the same manner as the essential oil itself.'

Germany, 2008. (1) Inhibitory effect of essential oils against herpes simplex HSV-2. In this trial, essential oils of **anise, thyme, ginger** and three other oils were pitted against herpes type 2, the virus responsible for most genital herpes infections. 'A clearly dose-dependent virucidal activity against HSV-2 could be demonstrated for all essential oils tested.' When HSV-2 was pre-treated with **thyme, ginger**, and one other of the oils, plaque formation was reduced by more than 90%. 'However, no inhibitory activity could be observed when the essential oils were added to the cells prior to infection with HSV-2... These results indicate that essential oils affected HSV-2 mainly before adsorption, probably by interacting with the viral envelope.'

Germany, 2008. (2). **Melissa** oil affects the infectivity of enveloped herpes viruses. The researchers put forward the argument that the herpes simplex virus might develop resistance to commonly used (pharmaceutical) agents. **Melissa** officinalis, also known as **lemon balm**, was examined, and its main constituents were identified. Next, the antiviral effect was quantified, with results of plaque formation 'significantly reduced by 98.8% for HSV-1 and 97.2% for HSV-2.' Overall results indicated that **melissa** oil affected the virus before adsorption, but not after penetration into the host cell – 'thus **lemon balm** is capable of exerting a direct antiviral effect on herpes viruses. And because of the lipophilic nature of **lemon balm** oil enabling skin penetration, '**melissa** might be suitable for topical treatment of herpetic infections.'

Germany/Iran, 2009. A research team, comprising virologists from Germany and Iran, set up a study to compare the antiviral action of three essential oils – **eucalyptus**, **tea tree** and **thyme** – to the major constituent from each of the three essential oils. The research referred to an earlier study where the anti-herpes activity of **eucalyptus**, **tea tree**, **thyme** and **manuka** oils had already been published. In this paper, aroma chemicals from **eucalyptus**, **tea tree** and **thyme** were tested against herpes simplex virus HSV-1. Using sufficient essential oil to damage or kill HSV-1 but staying at 'maximum non-cytotoxic concentrations', the three tested essential oils and most of the aroma chemicals (monoterpenes) under review 'were able to suppress viral infection by 80% to 96%.' 'These results suggest that the investigated drugs* directly inactivate the herpes virus and might interfere with virion envelope structures.' **Eucalyptus**, **tea tree** and **thyme** oil, along with some selected aromatic compounds, were tested. All essential oils and individual compounds exhibited an antiviral effect, with **tea tree** oil the most effective. When **tea tree** was tested in its natural form, it proved to have ten times higher results and lower toxicity than its isolated compounds.

*Essential oils are sometimes referred to as drugs in scientific research.

South Korea, 2018. The study was conducted to see whether essential oils had any antiviral activity against the influenza A virus – an enveloped RNA virus. As well as essential oils, the team analysed and tested some of the main aromatic compounds to determine whether there were any specific aromatic compounds associated with this activity. Over 60 essential oils were evaluated for antiviral activity against the influenza A virus. Laboratory trials demonstrated that only eleven of the tested essential oils had anti-influenza activity. Of the eleven antiviral essential oils, three were found to be potent antivirals. The other eight antiviral oils were not named in the published paper. The three potent antivirals – **marjoram, clary sage** and **aniseed** – exhibited high anti-influenza activity and were then analysed for their chemical composition, which was detected by GLC/MS analysis. It was found that the composition of aroma chemicals differed between the three oils except for linalool, which was detected in each. The three oils showing high anti-influenza activity had zero to low cytotoxicity in the concentration used in the experiment, which makes them ideal candidates for human use. However, persons with sensitive skin are sometimes allergic to linalool. As linalool was common to all three oils, the researchers suggest that this aroma chemical may have anti-influenza activity, but that 'further investigation is needed to characterise the antiviral activity of linalool against influenza A.' Latin names of the three named antiviral essential oils are thymus mastichina, salvia sclarea, pimpinella anisum.

Taiwan, 2020. This research is one of the first antiviral published papers to enter the public domain since the emergence of the coronavirus pandemic. With acknowledgement of a lack of antiviral medications for current use, along with the well known long and arduous process to bring a new drug to market, the objective of the Taiwanese research was to conduct computerised trials with already proven antiviral essential oils. The first stage was to look at the skin-safety aspects of thirty essential oils – known as cytotoxicity. Some major aroma compounds from essential oils, identified by GLC/MS analysis, were incorporated into the research.

Of the thirty essential oils investigated, just fifteen were chosen for the second research stage. These oils were non-cytotoxic, and therefore skin-safe – **geranium**, **eucalyptus**, **juniper**, **marjoram** and **tea tree** oils, among others, were not cytotoxic – up to a particular concentration. Some of the essential oils were found to be moderately cytotoxic; half a dozen essential oils were found to be highly cytotoxic. Overall, there were good results with **bergamot**, **eucalyptus**, **geranium**, **ginger**, **juniper**, **lavender**, **lemon**, **peppermint**, **rosemary** and **tea tree**. The essential oils of **geranium** and **lemon** were of most interest: their major components became a key part of the investigation. '**Geranium** oil represents a potent immune modulator and stimulates and cleanses the lymphatic system.' **Geranium** and **lemon** were trialled for specific action against the coronavirus – something that does not form any part of my book; however, these details can be found via the Citations. 'There is evidence to suggest that essential oils and their major components have displayed potent antiviral activity...yet, further studies are highly warranted to unveil the underlying molecular mechanisms of this inhibitory effect.' The research objective was to find effective essential oils that might be considered non-hazardous to epithelial cells. But that 'further studies are highly warranted to unveil the underlying molecular mechanisms.'

Turkey, 2012. A research team across five academic institutions investigated the antiviral activity of essential oils from a selection of plants in the family Umbelliferae and Labiatae. A series of tests were performed with a selection of essential oils against the herpes simplex virus (DNA) and parainfluenza virus (RNA). A comprehensive selection of essential oils and their individual compounds were investigated. Results showed that all essential oils and active constituents displayed varying inhibition against herpes simplex; some also had antiviral activity against the parainfluenza virus, notably **dill** and **peppermint**. Major individual chemicals from the essential oils were also part of the research – one of the key points was the discovery of the active molecules that make up the essential oils; in most cases, there are hundreds of molecules. And in conclusion, examples show how the terpene derivatives found in significant quantities in essential oils have the potential to affect the bioactivity of their respective essential oils. Therefore, the chemical composition of essential oils and the number of individual oil compounds are fundamental and relate to each other in terms of biological activity.'

Antiviral in silico research

Each of the research teams undertaking in silico research – from Algeria to the USA – have looked at the new virus responsible for Covid-19. Having an appreciation of past successful trials with essential oils and viruses, the international teams have then looked at the future potential of antiviral essential oils and or the individual components as a treatment for Covid-19.

Each team has published a scientific paper on their trials, selecting essential oils against herpes simplex HSV-1 and 2, influenza virus A, and other common viruses. With these results, university teams have – by computational methods – hypothesised essential oils and aromatic compounds as 'potentially useful as antiviral agents against SARS-CoV-2.' Although results were mixed, 'there is considerable evidence emerging from in vitro studies and trials for essential oils to be utilised as antiviral agents in the treatment of human viral infections.' These antiviral essential oils were mainly tested against enveloped RNA or DNA viruses such as herpes simplex virus type 1 and influenza A virus…as well as some non-enveloped.' 'There is evidence to suggest that essential oils and their major components have displayed potent antiviral activity to some coronaviruses… mainly through inhibition of viral replication.' In this section of my book, the objective is to bring to public attention a selection of meaningful work: and below, I attempt to précis the research: objectives, methods, and conclusions. Please bear in mind that the following proposals are purely hypothetical and cannot be assumed to be valid for human use until a considerable amount of further in vitro research has been undertaken.

Algeria, 2020. The research team acknowledges that the coronavirus: Covid-19 is causing havoc worldwide and that there are few antivirals on offer. 'Essential oils and their chemical constituents are known to be active against a wide range of viruses… Since the new strain of coronavirus, now named SARS-CoV-2, is still not completely understood, it is not yet possible to find which essential oils will offer the best level of protection.' 'More is learned about this virus on an almost weekly basis, but it could still be some considerable time before a cure is found. However, it is plausible to assume that some of the essential oils and related terpenes are likely to offer a measurable level of defence in the same way they do with many other known viruses.' The Algerian research team have included some interesting results regarding the mechanisms of antiviral activity. And I quote 'virucidal activity of essential oils, which are lipophilic by nature, is probably due to disruption of the viral membrane or interference with viral envelope proteins involved in host cell attachment. Since numerous essential oils have the ability to interrupt biological membranes, it follows that essential oils may also dislocate viral envelopes – an argument reinforced by electron micrographs of HSV-1 after **clove** oil (and one other oil); presented envelope interruption.'

Brazil, 2020. 'Essential oils have shown promise as antiviral agents against several pathogenic viruses' is the opening line of the introduction from the published research paper. Each university team working with essential oils and viruses will have a clear objective: to discover something new. 'In this work, we hypothesised that essential oil components may interact with key protein targets of Covid 19.' In this paper, the research team put forward the possibility that antiviral essential oils – with proven ability to kill or inhibit the growth of influenza viruses – could be utilised to control SARS-CoV-2 infection.' Molecular docking analysis was carried out using 171 essential oil components... each analysed for their potential use against a specific aspect of the coronavirus. This virtual research proved to be ineffective for the research purpose but concluded with the wording '...essential oil components may act synergistically...or they may provide some relief of Covid-19 symptoms.'

China, 2020. In this review, a two-person team studied in vitro antiviral research published within ten years, with the purpose to provide up-to-date information on the antiviral properties of essential oils. 'This review will provide and improve our understanding of the proper applications of essential oils in the future.' 'Plant-derived essential oils may serve as alternative sources of virus-induced disease therapy. Previous studies had demonstrated essential oils to be excellent candidates for treating antiviral-resistant infections associated with their chemical complexity, which confers broad-spectrum mechanisms of action and non-specific antiviral properties...well documented on a variety of viruses – influenza virus, HSV-1 and 2, HIV, yellow fever, avian influenza.' 'Antiviral studies in the past years focussed on enveloped viruses, while non-enveloped viruses have fewer active sites that the essential oils are able to target.' 'Essential oils interfere with free virions by modifying the virus envelope structure or masking the viral proteins which are necessary for viral adsorption and entry into the host cells.' 'Taken together, essential oils hold promise as candidates for prophylactic and therapeutic treatment of virus-induced diseases.' 'However, the mechanisms of action at the molecular level are inadequately elucidated, and plant sources investigated are relatively limited. Therefore, research in this regard deserves further attention.'

Ethiopia, 2014. The researchers looked at published papers documenting the antiviral activity of essential oils, tested against enveloped RNA and DNA viruses, such as herpes simplex virus type 1 and type 2 (DNA viruses), dengue virus type 2 (RNA virus), and influenza virus (RNA virus). 'However, two essential oils...were also tested against non-enveloped RNA and DNA viruses, such as adenovirus type 3 (DNA virus), poliovirus (RNA virus), and coxsackievirus group B (RNA virus). The nature, structural composition, and the functional groups present in the essential oils play an important role in determining the antimicrobial activity. Essential oils contain a variety of volatile molecules such as terpenes and terpenoids, phenol derived aromatic and aliphatic compounds, which might have bactericidal, virucidal, and fungicidal consequences. Essential oils directly affect the cell membrane of the pathogenic microorganism by causing an increase in permeability and leakage of vital intracellular constituents, disrupting the cell respiration and microbial enzyme system. Therefore, it has been suggested that the essential oils extracted from medicinal plants might be used as alternative antimicrobial natural substances, and play a great role in discovering new drugs.'

India, 2020. In this in silico work, university researchers only referenced in vitro trials with commonly available essential oils and their active compounds. The essential oils of interest included **rosemary**, **tea tree**, **bergamot**, clove, eucalyptus, melissa, peppermint and cinnamon. 'Inhalation of mentioned essential oils could be an adjuvant therapeutic strategy for Covid-19.' Of individual essential oils, the team had this to say about each essential oil: 'Bergamot. As the main volatile compounds in the oil show inhibitory action against influenza virus, the conclusion was that it may show inhibitory action against the SARS-CoV-2 virus.' Eucalyptus. Research referred to in the vapour phase, found that it was effective against the influenza virus. And like rosemary oil, eucalyptus contains 1,8-cineol... 'Therefore, it is believed it will show vigorous activity against the Covid-19 virus.' Tea tree oil. 'Active components of tea tree oil showed strong antiviral activity' and 'all these properties suggested the probability of the effectiveness of tea tree oil against Covid-19.' Peppermint oil. 'In vitro trials have demonstrated noteworthy antimicrobial and antiviral action.' Cinnamon oil. 'Its active components show strong antiviral activity.' Melissa. Because of its active constituents, lemon balm (melissa) essential oil shows inhibitory activity against the influenza virus, and its active constituents can arrest the replication cycle of influenza virus.' 'Because of its antiviral activity, it could be used in treatment against Covid-19.' The paper concluded with the statement 'whether these oils are effective against coronavirus or not, will need clinical trials.' 'But all these mentioned oils can definitely be used to stop further growth and get some relief from the deadly virus.'

Nigeria, 2020. The title of the paper 'exploring essential oils as prospective therapy against the ravaging coronavirus SARS-CoV-2,' looks at essential oils that have demonstrated virucidal properties with advantages of low toxicity. Over 70% of medicinal drugs have a natural origin or were motivated by natural product chemistry, and natural products…and, over time, have delivered up to 40% of the present antibacterial, antifungal, antiviral or anticancer molecules for the pharmaceutical industry.' 'The pharmaceutical industry is increasingly targeting volatile constituents of medicinal plants with the aim of identifying lead compounds, focussing mainly on suitable alternative antiviral agents. In recent years there has been a growing interest in the use of medicinal plants.' 'Aromatic plants produce a diversity of chemical constituents with potential to inhibit viral replication and chemical molecules from natural products.' Essential oils contain the following (primary) classes of aroma chemicals: Terpenes. Esters. Alcohols. Phenols. Aldehydes. 'Essential oils are among the plant-derived antiviral molecules that are employed in phytomedicine. They prevent the replication of some viruses such as HIV, herpes simplex, and severe acute human respiratory diseases.' 'In a study conducted by Wen et al, a total of 221 phytochemical constituents were tested for antiviral effect against SARS-CoV. 'Some of these phytochemical constituents of essential oils were revealed for the first time to display specific and significant anti-SARS-CoV effect and thus offer a new pathway for improvement of anti-SARS-CoV drugs.' In conclusion, 'the information presented provides a basis for reviving the old art of 'essential oil therapy' based on our modern scientific knowledge of the mechanism of action. Thus, essential oils and their constituents can hopefully be considered in the future for more clinical assessment and possible applications in the search for vaccines against the ravaging coronavirus.'

Pakistan, 2020. This research paper began with the phrase, 'essential oils have long been known to have anti-inflammatory, immunomodulatory, bronchodilatory, and antiviral properties and are being proposed to have activity against SARS-CoV-2 virus.' 'Owing to their lipophilic nature, essential oils are advocated to penetrate viral membranes, easily leading to membrane disruption.' 'Moreover, essential oils contain multiple active phytochemicals that can act synergistically on multiple stages of viral replication and induce positive effects on the host respiratory system.' 'At present, only computer-aided docking and a few in vitro studies are available which show the anti-SARS-CoV-2 activities of essential oils.' 'Once the virus gains entry into the respiratory tract, SARS-CoV-2 causes damage to the epithelial cells of the airways, making lungs unable to clear mucus, which can lead to pneumonia.' 'Numerous researchers have studied the antibacterial, antifungal, antioxidant, and antiviral properties of essential oils. Essential oils are known to be active against a wide variety of viruses.' Oils mentioned include **tea tree** and **manuka**, among others, as they 'were found to inhibit the ineffective ability of some viruses, indicating the immense antiviral potential of essential oils.' '**Eucalyptus** oil reported having in vitro antiviral activity against various strains of viruses including mumps, herpes simplex viruses and influenza A viruses.' 'Having established the antiviral activity of **eucalyptus** oil and its main components against respiratory viruses, multiple researchers have attempted to explore the antiviral efficacy of **eucalyptus** oil against SARS, using in vitro assays and molecular docking techniques.' Having put forward the future potential of essential oils to tackle severe viral infection, the conclusion states, 'the existing information about these essential oils is very preliminary, and the majority of claims are based on data obtained from computer-aided docking and preliminary in vitro studies. In this regard, well-planned in vitro and in vivo studies are warranted to establish the safe dose and clinical efficacy of essential oils...to combat this viral disorder and its associated complications.'

USA, 2016. This in silico paper, references several in vitro tests from previously published research papers that prove the antiviral capabilities of essential oils. For many years asserted to be an alternative treatment option for influenza infections, the following essential oils have shown anti-influenza virus activity – **bergamot**, **cinnamon leaf**, **eucalyptus**, **geranium**, **lavender**, **lemongrass**, **tea tree** and **thyme**. This research refers to 104 published papers – some in silico and others in vitro. Many of these papers looked at the mode of action of essential oils and their potential future use in the management of influenza pandemics. Essential oils and their individual constituents were assessed regarding their antiviral activity against the influenza A virus. **Bergamot** oil was 'shown to demonstrate in vitro anti-influenza activity – 100% inhibition of type A at low concentration.' '**Cinnamon leaf** oil showed 100% in vitro inhibition of influenza type A at...100% inhibition after 30 minutes exposure to the vapour.' '**Eucalyptus** oil – mainly the commonly available **eucalyptus globulus** – was referenced in a number of previously published papers as a 90% inhibitor of influenza type A virus. '**Geranium** essential oil has shown 80% in vitro inhibition of influenza A at low concentration.' '**Lemongrass** essential oil showed 100% inhibition of influenza A at a low concentration.' '**Tea tree** oil showed 100% inhibition of influenza type A virus at low concentration.' 'Essential oil of **thyme** proved to have 100% inhibition of influenza type A virus at low concentration.' In conclusion 'essential oils have shown promise in the prevention and treatment of influenza infections, corroborating much of the traditional medicinal use of the corresponding plants. In addition to their antiviral activities, many of the essential oils can also relieve some of the symptoms of influenza. There are many opportunities for additional research on antiviral essential oils...with respect to influenza infection.'

Membrane disruption research

Ever since essential oils have been used for the treatment of diseases, both human and animal, there has been speculation as to the exact ways in which viruses and bacteria become overpowered by an essential oil, with the vague term 'disinfectant' the generally accepted descriptive. The big question "How do essential oils disrupt bacterial cell walls and viral membranes?" has largely been unexplored. But what is well known among people who use essential oils, is that some have the ability to penetrate the plastic cap of an essential oil bottle if left unopened for a long time, perhaps because of a personal dislike of the aroma. Common sense would suggest that if essential oils are capable of penetrating hard plastic, then they ought to be able to damage a bacterial cell wall or viral membrane. Today, we have evidence of the membrane disrupting qualities of some essential oils, and over the following pages I have précised research from ten universities – from 1995 to 2021 – proving the term 'antiviral' to be justified. Each essential oil is composed of aromatic hydrocarbons (most commonly monoterpenes) and depending on the aromatic plant, any of the following – phenols, alcohols, esters, aldehydes, ketones and oxides. Essential oils do not discriminate between bacteria and viruses so, although the following research is mainly with bacteria, some university research teams have concluded that the mode of action of an essential oil will be the same for viruses as it is for bacteria.

For ease of reading, I have used the name of the lead researcher and year of publication, which I find an interesting way to follow the individual approaches of each research team. Full details of the published papers can be found in Citations.

Sikkema et al, 1995. 'The metabolic pathways of various aromatics...were studied. The toxicity of these aromatic compounds to microorganisms is important...but not many researchers have studied the mechanism of this toxic action. In this review, we present general ideas derived from the various reports mentioning toxic effects. Most importantly, lipophilic hydrocarbons accumulate in the membrane lipid bilayer, affecting the structural and functional properties of these membranes. As a result of accumulated hydrocarbon molecules, the membrane loses its integrity, and an increase in permeability... has been observed in several instances.'

Cox et al, 2000. 'Melaleuca alternifolia (tea tree) is well known for its broad-spectrum antimicrobial activity and this research was to find its mode of action using a range of investigative methods. Exposure of Gram-negative and Gram-positive organisms to minimum inhibitory concentrations of tea tree oil, it was observed that tea tree oil inhibited respiration and increased permeability of membranes...and also caused potassium ion leakage. The ability of tea tree oil to disrupt the permeability of cell membrane structures...is the most likely source of its lethal action.'

Trombetta et al, 2005. It is because essential oils merge readily with fats and oils, that essential oils – or their constituent parts – are able to cause 'membrane expansion, increased membrane fluidity and permeability, inhibition of respiration and alteration of ion transport processes.' Three essential oil components – menthol, thymol, and linalyl acetate – were evaluated for their ability to damage bio membranes. 'Lipid constituents of a cell membrane... provide the membrane with its barrier function and play a role in a variety of processes in the bacterial cell.' 'Results obtained allow us to speculate that the antimicrobial activity of the terpenes under investigation may be caused, at least partially, by their penetration into... lipids' and consequently to cause an alteration of the fatty parts of plasma membranes, 'resulting in alterations of membrane permeability and in leakage of intracellular materials.' The paper concludes with the wording 'furthermore, the drugs might cross the cell membranes, penetrating the interior of the cell and interacting with intracellular sites critical for antibacterial activity.'

Cristani et al, 2007. Trombetta was one of the team in this research. The objective was to challenge the antimicrobial efficacy of four monoterpenes – carvacrol, thymol, p-cymene and gamma-terpinene, against three different types of bacteria and ... to obtain a better understanding of their mechanism of action; and damage caused to bio membranes by these four monoterpenes was evaluated. The published paper concluded 'our findings lead us to speculate that the antimicrobial effect of the four aroma chemicals tested may result, partially at least, from a significant alteration to a part of the membrane.'

Heipieper et al, 2010. 'Several classes of organic compounds are toxic for living organisms as they accumulate in and disrupt cell membranes. The toxic effect of most hydrocarbons is caused by general, nonspecific effects on membrane fluidity due to their accumulation in the lipid bilayer; exceptions are hydrocarbons with specific chemically active functional groups... that show an additional chemical toxicity.'

Ocazionez et al, 2010. 'The inhibitory effect of the essential oil seems to cause direct virus inactivation before adsorption on host cell.' The precise mechanism of the virucidal action of essential oils is still not fully understood. Results of the studies evaluating the interference of the essential oil on steps of the viral infection cycle, indicate that the inhibitory effect occurs during adsorption and penetration steps but not after penetration of the virus into the cell. One could speculate that components present in the oil interfere with the virion envelope structures...masking viral proteins which are necessary for adsorption and entry into the host cell. The main components of the essential oils tested in this study were monoterpenes, including carvone, geranial, neral and limonene. 'The in vitro replication abilities of the herpes simplex virus HSV-1, hepatitis B virus and HIV human immunodeficiency virus were suppressed by the previous exposure to essential oils but not by treatment of the cell with the essential oil before the adsorption of the virus.' The present paper has demonstrated the inhibitory effect of the essential oil of Lippia citriodora...and seems to penetrate the skin and might act inside the cell to block viral replication.'The inhibitory effect of Lippia citriodora essential oil on dengue virus serotypes replication was investigated. Antiviral activity was defined as the concentration of essential oil that caused 50% reduction of the virus plaque. No viral inhibitory effect was observed by addition of the essential oil after virus adsorption. The inhibitory effect of the essential oil seems to cause direct virus inactivation before adsorption on host cell.'

Ma et al, 2020. 'Essential oils interfere with free virions by modifying virus envelope structure...necessary for viral adsorption and entry into the host cells. (A virion is an entire virus particle).'

Wink, 2020. 'Many plants produce secondary metabolites (PSMs) which have antiviral activities. Among the antiviral PSMs, lipophilic terpenoids in essential oils can disturb the lipid envelope of viruses... attack viral proteins present in the viral membrane or inside the virus particle... Both phenolics and essential oils are active against free viral particles but not, or to a lesser degree, after a virus has entered a host cell. Owing to the lipophilic nature of essential oils, there is the potential for an essential oil component to enter into the lipid layer of a viral envelope, affecting fluidity and often rupturing the membranes.'

Sharma et al, 2020. 'The present in silico study was designed to evaluate the effect of Eucalyptol (1,8 cineole) an essential oil component from eucalyptus oil.'

Reference was made to another research paper. 'Data obtained showed that 1,8-cineole (eucalyptol from eucalyptus) can bind with a viral particle and inhibit viral reproduction.' Conclusions: 'Therefore, eucalyptol may represent potential treatment to act as COVID-19 Mpro inhibitor. However, further research is necessary to investigate their potential medicinal use.'

Yap et al, 2021. 'The complex mixture of essential oils usually shows a higher antiviral activity than individual compounds. Different mechanisms of antiviral activity of different essential oils and their constituents seem to be present. The antiviral activity of the essential oil is principally due to direct virucidal effects (by denaturing viral structural proteins). Proposed mechanisms suggest that essential oils interfere with the virus envelope by inhibiting specific processes in the viral replication cycle or by masking viral components, which are necessary for adsorption or entry into host cells, thus, they prevent the cell-to-cell virus diffusion.'

CITATIONS
Antiviral in vitro research

Canada
Anti-influenza virus activity of essential oils and vapours. Vimalanathan S, et al. Dept of pathology and laboratory medicine, University of British Columbia, Vancouver, Canada. Published 2014, American Journal of Essential Oils and Natural Products.

Germany
Antiviral activity of Australian tea tree oil and eucalyptus oil against herpes simplex virus in cell culture. Schnitzler P, et al. Department of Virology, Hygiene Institute, University of Heidelberg, Germany. Published 2001, International Journal of Phytotherapy & Phytopharmacology.

Virucidal effect of peppermint oil on the enveloped viruses herpes simplex virus type 1 and type 2 in vitro. Schumacher A, et al. Department of Virology, Hygiene Institute, Faculty of Medicine, University of Heidelberg, Heidelberg, Germany. Published 2003, International Journal of Phytotherapy & Phytopharmacology.

Virucidal activity of a beta-triketone-rich essential oil of Leptospermum scoparium (manuka oil) against HSV-1 and HSV-2 in cell culture. Reichling J, et al. Institute of Pharmacy and Molecular Biotechnology, Department of Biology, University of Heidelberg, Heidelberg, Germany. Published 2005, Planta Med.

Inhibitory effect of essential oils against herpes simplex virus type 2. Koch C, et al. Department of Virology, Hygiene Institute, University of Heidelberg, Heidelberg, Germany. Published 2008, Phytomedicine: International Journal of Phytotherapy & Phytopharmacology.

Melissa officinalis oil affects infectivity of enveloped herpesviruses. Schnitzler P, Schuhmacher A, Astani A, Reichling J. Department of Virology, Hygiene Institute, University of Heidelberg, Germany. Published 2008, Phytomedicine.

Germany/Iran
Comparative study on the antiviral activity of selected monoterpenes derived from essential oils. Astani A, et al. Dept of Virology, Hygiene Institute, University of Heidelberg, Germany; Dept of Biology, Institute of

Pharmacy and Molecular Biotechnology, University of Heidelberg, Germany; Yazd Shahid Sadoghi University of Medical Science, Iran. Published 2010, Phytotherapy Research, Wiley.

South Korea
Chemical constituents of essential oils possessing anti-influenza A/WS/33 virus activity. Choi H, et al. Dept of Beauty Science, Kwangju Women's University, Kwangju, S. Korea. Published Nov 2018, Korea Centres for Disease Control and Prevention.

Taiwan
Geranium and lemon essential oils and their active compounds down regulate angiotensin-converting enzyme t2 (ACE2), a SARS-CoV-2 spike receptor-binding domain, epithelial cells. Kumar K, et al. Department of Forestry, National Chung Hsing University, Taichung 402, Taiwan. Published June 2020, Plants.

Turkey

Antimicrobial and antiviral effects of essential oils from selected ...plants and individual essential oil components. Orhan E, et al. Dept of Pharmacognosy, Faculty of Pharmacy, Gazi University, Ankara, Turkey; Pharmacognosy and Pharmaceutical Botany Unit, Faculty of Pharmacy, Eastern Mediterranean University, Turkish Republic of Northern Cypress; Dept of Pharmaceutical Microbiology, Faculty of Pharmacy, Gazi University, Ankara, Turkey; Dept of Field Crops, Faculty of Agriculture, Selcuk University, Konya, Turkey. Published Dec 2009, Turkish Journal of Biology.

Antiviral in silico research

Algeria

Effective anti-viral activity of essential oils and their characteristic terpenes against coronaviruses: an update. Boukhatem M, et al. Dept Biologie et Physiologie Cellulaire, Faculte des Sciences de la Nature et de la Vie, Université Blida, Algeria. Published 2020, Journal of Pharmacology & Clinical Toxicology.

Brazil
Essential oils as anti-viral agents, potential of essential oils to treat SARS-COV-2 Infection: An in silico Investigation. da Silva J K, et al. Laboratorio de Biotecnologia de Enzima e Biotransformacoes, Universidade Federal do Para. Belem PA 66075-900, BRAZIL. Published 2020, International Journal of Molecular Science.

China
Antiviral effects of plant derived essential oils and their components: an updated review. Ma L, et al. R&D Center for Aromatic Plants, Shanghai Jiao Tong University, Shanghai, China. Published 2020, Molecules.

Ethiopa
Antimicrobial activity of essential oils extracted from medicinal plants against the pathogenic microorganisms. Akthar M, et al. Department of Biology, College of Natural Sciences, Jimma University, Ethiopia. Department of Plant Science, College of Agriculture and Veterinary Sciences, Ambo University, Ambo 19, Ethiopia. Published 2014, Biological Sciences and Pharmaceutical Research.

India
Inhalation of essential oils: could be adjuvant therapeutic strategy for Covid-19. Patne T, et al. Institute of Pharmaceutical Sciences and Research, Pimpri, Pune, Maharashtra, India. Published 2020, Journal of Pharmaceutical Sciences & Research.

Nigeria
Exploring essential oils as prospective therapy against the ravaging coronavirus SARS-CoV-2. Ojah E, et al. Medicinal Chemistry Research Group, organic chemistry unit, Department of Chemistry, University of Ibadan, Ibadan, Nigeria. Published 2020, Ibero-American Journal of Medicine.

Pakistan
Covid 19 and therapy with essential oils having anti-viral, anti-inflammatory, and immunomodulatory properties. Asif M, et al. Dept of Pharmacology, Faculty of Pharmacy, The Islamia University of Bahawalpur, Pakistan. Published 2020, Springer Nature, Switzerland.

USA

Essential oils as complementary and alternative medicines for the treatment of influenza. Setzer W. Department of Chemistry, University of Alabama, Alabama, USA Published 2016, American Journal of Essential Oils and Natural Products.

Membrane disruption research

Mechanisms of membrane toxicity of hydrocarbons. Sikkema J, et al. Department of Food Science, Wageningen Agricultural University, The Netherlands. Published 1995, Microbiological Reviews.

The mode of antimicrobial action of the essential oil of melaleuca alternifolia (tea tree oil). Cox S D, et al. Centre for Biostructural and Biomolecular Research, University of Western Sydney, Hawkesbury, New South Wales, Western Australia. Published 2000, Journal of Applied Microbiology.

Mechanisms of antibacterial action of three monoterpenes. Trombetta D, et al. University of Messina, Italy. Published 2005, Antimicrobial Agents Chemotherapy.

Interaction of four monoterpenes contained in essential oils with model membranes: implications for their antibacterial activity. Cristani M, et al. University of Messina, Italy. Published 2007, Journal of Agricultural and Food Chemistry.

Virucidal activity of Colombian *Lippia* essential oils on dengue virus replication in vitro. Ocazionez R, et al. Laboratorio de Arbovirus, Centro de Investigaciones en Enfermedades Tropicales, Universidad Industrial de Santander, Bucaramanga, Colombia. Published 2010, Memórias do Instituto Oswaldo Cruz.

Toxicity of hydrocarbons to microorganisms. Heipieper H, et al. Department of Bioremediation, Helmholtz Centre for Environmental Research—UFZ, Leipzig, Germany. Published 2010, Springer: Handbook of Hydrocarbon and Lipid Microbiology.

Potential of DNA intercalating alkaloids and other plant secondary metabolites against SARS-CoV-2 causing Covid-19. Wink M. Institute of Pharmacy and Molecular Biotechnology, Heidelberg University, Germany. Published 2020, Diversity.

Antiviral effects of plant-derived essential oils and their components: an updated review. Ma L, et al. R&D Center for Aromatic Plants, Shanghai Jiao Tong University, Shanghai 200240, China; Dept of Landscape Architecture, Shanghai Jiao Tong University, Shanghai, China. Published 2020, Molecules.

Eucalyptol (1,8 cineole) from eucalyptus essential oil a potential inhibitor of COVID 19 corona virus infection by Molecular docking studies. Sharma A, et al. Dept of Biotechnology, Lyallpur Khalsa College Jalandhar, India. Published 2020, Preprints.

Membrane disruption properties of essential oils—a double-edged sword? Yap P, et al. Jeffrey Cheah School of Medicine and Health Sciences, Monash University, Malaysia. Published 2021, MDPI, Basel, Switzerland.

https://longitudeprize.org is a website I recommend checking out, as antimicrobial resistance (AMR) is a serious health concern threatening the future of post surgical survival. The **longitude prize** site seeks to educate the general public about the dangers of the overuse of antibiotics.

GLOSSARY

Adsorption. The meaning of adsorption refers to the process by which a chemical reaction creates a thin film to coat a surface. Not to be confused with absorption.

Airborne. The coronavirus is airborne as it is lighter than air. Although in the early days of coronavirus, we were told that 'droplets' were responsible for the transmission of the virus, it was eventually acknowledged that the virus was airborne.

Alternative medicine. A remedy or a way of treating a disease or ailment with natural products – herbs, essential oils, vitamins and minerals. Or physical therapies such as acupuncture or massage. Treatments that doctors do not prescribe.

Anti-depressant. Generally, a term used to refer to a drug with SSRI properties. In this book, the term anti-depressant denotes the therapeutic properties of some essential oils. Unlike SSRIs, essential oils are not taken orally but work by means of massaging diluted essential oils into the skin or by inhaling the vapours.

Anti-inflammatory. In orthodox medicine, anti-inflammatory drugs such as paracetamol are prescribed to relieve pain, redness and heat – the classic manifestations of the inflammatory process. In this book, the term anti-inflammatory refers essential oils with the ability to reduce heat, pain or swelling.

Antimicrobial. A drug – whether natural or from a pharmaceutical company – that can kill or stop the growth of microbes. Bacteria, fungi, viruses, parasitic infections are all microbial.

Antimicrobial resistance. When microbes evolve over time to evade being killed by antibiotics.

Antibiotic. Drugs prescribed to treat or prevent many types of bacterial infections. Antibiotics work by killing bacteria or preventing them from spreading but should never be taken for any viral disease as antibiotics don't kill viruses but will damage the immune system.

Antibodies. Substances that are produced by the body's immune system to identify and neutralise foreign objects such as pathogenic bacteria and viruses.

Antidote. An antidote is a drug or chemical that counteracts (neutralises) the effects of a poison or a drug that has caused harm to a patient.

Antioxidant. Something that fights free radicals in your body is known as an antioxidant. Free radicals can cause harm if levels become high, as these have been linked to severe diseases.

Antispasmodic. Generally, a drug used to relieve spasms of involuntary muscles. Some essential oils are antispasmodic. One example is peppermint oil.

Avian influenza. Avian flu is a disease of birds and fowl and is also known as bird flu.

Anxiety. Anxiety is what we feel when we are worried, tense or afraid – particularly about things that are about to happen or which we think could happen in the future. Anxiety is fear and apprehension about what will happen next. But when anxiety becomes chronic – for whatever reason – it causes an unhappy, tense feeling that damages the body and can disrupt sleep, work, and relationships.

Autoimmune disease. When the body senses danger from a virus or other infection, the immune system kicks into gear to attack what it regards as NON-SELF, but occasionally some healthy cells get caught up in this response, causing the immune system to attack human cells that are SELF and not meant to be attacked.

Bacterial membrane. A bacterial membrane is a selective permeability barrier that regulates the passage of substances into and out of the cell.

Bactericidal. Cidal means to kill. Bactericide means to kill bacteria.

Big Pharma. See pharmaceutical.

Biome. A biome is a regional or global biotic community, such as grassland or desert. In the human body, the microbiome – often shortened to the biome – is an integral part of the immune system and digestive system. One of its functions is to protect humans against germs. The human biome is the body's healthy bacteria and is easily damaged by antibiotics.

Blisters. A common blister is caused on the feet after constant rubbing by the wearing of inappropriate footwear. The top layers of skin get separated from the underlying layers by the body's protective liquid – lymph. Blisters can also be caused by a virus – for example, herpes simplex of the lips or inside the mouth.

Botanical. A word that refers to anything to do with plants. Botanical medicine or phytomedicine would be a medicine made from a plant.

Brain Fog. Confusion, forgetfulness and a lack of focus and mental clarity. This condition can be caused by overworking, lack of sleep, stress or recovery from a debilitating illness. It is not a medical or scientific term. It is a condition experienced by many people during and after cancer therapies and is now prevalent among people suffering from long Covid.

Bronchodilator. A drug that causes widening of the bronchi, for example, an inhaled drug for the alleviation of asthma. Essential oils of lavender, eucalyptus and tea tree reduce inflammation of the airways in people with asthma.

Capillaries. As part of the circulatory system, capillaries are the smallest conduits of oxygenated blood, reaching the fingertips, facial skin and scalp. When capillaries become damaged, there is less oxygen being transported to peripheral areas of the body.

Cardio Pulmonary Resuscitation/CPR. A lifesaving technique that's useful in many emergencies such as heart attacks or near-drowning.

Chemotherapy. Powerful drugs given to cancer patients in the hope of killing cancer cells and saving lives. Unfortunately, chemotherapy drugs also destroy other fast-growing cells – of the immune system, hair and fingernails.

Chronic fatigue syndrome. A complex disorder characterised by extreme fatigue that lasts for at least six months and has not been linked to any specific underlying medical condition. Fatigue worsens with physical or mental activity but doesn't improve with rest. CFS is the same as Myalgic Encephalomyelitis, often shortened to M.E. With no cure, CFS sufferers often look to vitamins and aromatherapy for help.

Chronic insomnia. An inability to fall asleep or after falling asleep to wake up and be unable to return to sleep. A lack of sufficient sleep, experienced regularly, is a problem, as sound sleep is necessary for a healthy immune system and sound mental judgement.

Circulatory system. The body system that circulates blood and lymph through the body, consisting of the heart, blood vessels, blood, lymph, and lymphatic vessels and glands.

Cold sore. A sore that develops into a blister on the lips (and sometimes inside the cheeks) due to infection with HSV-1 herpes simplex virus. Genital sores are caused by infection with the HSV-2 herpes simplex virus.

Colostrum. A nutrient-rich fluid produced by women immediately after giving birth that is loaded with immune, growth and tissue repair factors. It is a complex biological fluid that helps in the development of immunity in the newborn by acting as a natural antimicrobial agent to stimulate the maturation of an infant's immune system.

Compress/Foot Compress. A compress consists of a pad of lint or other absorbent material pressed on to part of the body to relieve inflammation, regulate temperature or stop bleeding. Hot or cold water can be used for a compress. A cold compress with a few drops of lavender oil makes an effective forehead compress to help relieve a fever or headache.

Intensive care units. These are hospital-based urgent care facilities where a patient requires a lot of attention, such as following heart surgery, a serious accident or a powerful infection: anything that is life-threatening. Critical Care Unit is the US term for an ICU – intensive care unit.

Cytotoxic. Non-cytotoxic. Cytotoxic is a substance that is toxic to living cells. A few essential oils are cytotoxic and should not be used for massage. Non-cytotoxic essential oils have been proven safe on the skin and listed as GRAS. GRAS stands for Generally Regarded As Safe.

DNA. The shortened form of Deoxyribonucleic Acid. Viruses are either DNA or RNA.

Dermal irritation. A term used to describe the effect of specific essential oils on the skin. Essential oils known to be dermal irritants should not be used on the skin.

Enveloped and Non-Enveloped viruses. A virus is either enveloped or non-enveloped. Enveloped viruses are in a lipid membrane. Non-enveloped viruses do not have a lipid covering, but their effects on humans can be just as devastating. These "naked" viruses only need their protein-based capsid and host detector proteins to infect host cells.

Endemic. Epidemic. Pandemic. Disease is endemic if it is restricted to a particular geographical area. An epidemic is when a disease spreads quickly through a town, city or country. A pandemic is when a disease has spread around the world.

Epithelial Membrane/Epithelial cells. The epithelium is a type of body tissue that forms the covering on your body's internal and external surfaces. Mucous membranes in the nose are nasal epithelial cells where the inhaled SARS-CoV-2 virus binds and starts replicating.

Febrifuge. A medicine used to reduce fever. Paracetamol is common in general medicine, whereas eucalyptus is used in alternative medicine.

Fringe medicine. See alternative medicine.

Fumigation. The action or process of disinfecting or purifying a specific building area with fumes of certain chemicals. As essential oils are nature's chemicals, they can be used to fumigate a room – in the home or in a hospital setting to kill viruses.

Gram-Negative and Gram-Positive. Terms that differentiate the two types of bacteria. A broad-spectrum antibiotic is designed to kill both types of bacteria.

Herpes Simplex HSV-1. A viral infection of the lips and mouth. Occasionally the eyes are affected. See also Cold Sores.

Herpes Simplex HSV-2. A viral infection of the genitals.

HIV. While HIV is a virus that may cause an infection, AIDS (short for acquired immunodeficiency syndrome) is a condition.

Hydrophobic. Essential oils are hydrophobic, meaning that they do not dissolve in water.

Hypersensitive. Skin hypersensitivity is characterised by discomfort and profound sensitivity to household products or skin products.

IBS. Irritable bowel syndrome is a common condition affecting the digestive system.

Jojoba. A liquid wax from the seed of the jojoba plant (Simmondsia Chinensis), a shrub native to the deserts of North America.

Lesion (Pustular). Pustules are small lesions filled with pus. They're typically the result of acne, boils, or impetigo but can also result from a severe infection with herpes simplex virus.

Lipid membrane. A substance like fats and oils form a double-layered surface of cells.

Lipophilic. Essential oils are lipophilic, meaning that they dissolve well in fats.

Melatonin. A hormone primarily released by the pineal gland at night that has long been associated with control of the sleep-wake cycle.

Membrane disruption. Membrane disruption and permeation are actions in the eradication of a microorganism – such as a virus.

Metabolic. The chemical reaction in the body's cells that converts food into energy – that we know as metabolism.

MRSA. Methicillin-resistant Staphylococcus aureus. The first of many antibiotic-resistant bacteria.

Mucous membranes. Membranes line the body cavities that lead to the outside of the body, such as the respiratory, digestive, and urogenital tracts. Mucous membranes all have a surface layer of epithelial cells.

ME (Myalgic Encephalomyelitis). see Chronic Fatigue Syndrome.

Nasal-stomach tube. A nasogastric tube is a flexible rubber or plastic tube that is passed through the nose, down through the oesophagus and into the stomach.

Neonatal. Neonatal means newborn. Newborn healthy babies go home with the mother a day or two after birth. Premature babies or poorly babies would be cared for in a neonatal ward.

Nervous energy. Nervous energy results from having more than the usual amounts of cortisol and adrenaline in the body, generally due to a stressful situation.

Nervous tension. Feeling anxious and tense and having a sense of impending danger, panic or doom.

OTC. Over The Counter. An OTC medicine may be purchased from a pharmacy without a prescription.

Paediatrician. The title of a medical practitioner specialising in children and their diseases.

Palliative Care. Non-medical care for people nearing the end of their lives, when nothing more can be done to save them. Palliative care is commonly used for cancer patients.

Parainfluenza. Human parainfluenza viruses (HPIVs) commonly cause upper and lower respiratory infections, including colds, bronchitis, croup, and pneumonia. It is not related to influenza (the flu).

Pathogen. A pathogen is something that causes disease. A germ can be any one of – bacteria, viruses, fungi. Anything that is disease-causing is known as pathogenic.

Pathology. The study of pathogens.

Permeability. A substance – such as soil, sand, fabric etc. that allows fluids to pass through.

Pharmaceutical. Big Pharma refers to large pharmaceutical companies. The pharmaceutical industry discovers, develops, produces and markets drugs for use as medications, with the aim to cure, vaccinate or alleviate symptoms.

Pharmacology. The study of pharmaceutical drugs.

Phytomedicine. The science of medicines from plants. Essential oils, when used for therapeutic purposes, come under the heading of Phytomedicine.

Plant Derivative. Plant-derived compounds, including those extracted from essential oils.

Plaque assay reduction. The plaque assay is a well-established method for measuring virus concentration.

Post Traumatic Stress Disorder. PTSD is an anxiety disorder that results from very stressful, frightening or distressing events.

Prognosis. A medical opinion of the likely course of a medical condition.

Pustular Matter. The thick fluid containing dead tissue after an infection that has caused blisters is eventually expelled.

RNA. The short form of Ribonucleic acid.

SARS-CoV-2. Severe Acute Respiratory Syndrome (Coronavirus) that appeared in 2019. SARS-CoV-1 occurred in 2003.

Solar plexus. Part of the sympathetic nervous system, the solar plexus plays a vital role in the functioning of the stomach, kidneys, liver and adrenal glands.

Strep throat. Strep throat is an infection caused by streptococcus bacteria.

Systemic. Relating to the entire body rather than a single system such as the respiratory system.

Systemic neonatal herpes. Neonatal herpes is a herpes infection in a young baby and, when systemic, can quickly become fatal.

Topical therapeutic use. When diluted essential oils are applied to the skin for a therapeutic purpose and generally administered via massage.

Toxic. A toxic substance that is poisonous to one degree or another.

Vaporised. When an essential oil or blend of essential oils is turned into vapour form by adding drops to a diffuser, putting a few drops into a mug/bowl of hot water, or even leaving the top off a bottle of an essential oil. It is when the aromatic liquid diffuses into the air.

Virus. A virus is a small collection of genetic code, either DNA or RNA. A virus cannot replicate alone and must infect host cells to make copies of itself.

Viral load. The amount of virus in an infected person.

Viral protein. Non-enveloped viruses (naked viruses) are encased in protein.

Virion envelope. A viral envelope.

Virion. The entire virus particle.

Virology. The study of viruses.

Virucidal. A chemical or drug that is capable of killing a virus.

Virulence. The severity or harmfulness of a disease.

Virus inactivation. When a virus is prevented from replicating by its removal or rendering it non-infectious.

Viscosity. The thickness of an oil. Some essential oils, such as lemon and bergamot, are non-viscous. A few essential oils, such as sandalwood, are viscous.

Visual problems. Covid-19 can cause visual issues when the eyes become sensitive to light; there is a pain in the eye socket; when there is difficulty in focussing or there is blurred vision.

Volatile oil. A term given to essential oils. Volatile is something that is unstable. Essential oils are first liquid but become vapours when evaporated into the air. Volatile oils are flammable and should be kept away from naked flames.

Zoonotic. A disease that can be transmitted from an animal to a human or from a human to an animal.

BIOGRAPHY

Maggie was one of the first published authors on the subject of aromatherapy in the English language when Harper Collins (Thorsons) published *Aromatherapy for Women* in 1985. The book has been re-published several times, in many languages, and with international sales, has sold more than 700,000 copies. In 2022, *Antiviral Aromatherapy* has been written and published for anyone interested in taking an alternative look at getting well and staying well.

Maggie grew up in West London, and as a child, would gather rose petals from her neighbours' front gardens. She loved the scent and rubbed her dolls with the fragrant juice 'to make them feel better' – but Maggie never imagined that many years later, a massage with essential oil of rose would be known as aromatherapy. Since losing her father at the age of 14, Maggie was determined to make her own way in life, being as independent as possible while always hoping to find the perfect job – one that would be fulfilling. Maggie was twenty-one when she discovered library books on the subject of natural healing and quickly became passionate about the ability to utilise gentle remedies instead of pharmaceuticals. In 1972, Maggie knew alternative medicine was going to become her life's work, and it was that passion that brought her into contact with Robert Tisserand (now an author and international lecturer on the subject of aromatherapy). The eleven-year marriage produced three beautiful children, and Maggie utilised essential oils during pregnancy, childbirth and child-rearing – watching them grow up healthy and strong, without antibiotics or pain killers and away from the doctors' surgery.

Essential oils – an integral part of Maggie's life – inspired her to write a book based on her personal experiences, as friends would regularly ring her for advice. In 1983, when based in Brighton, Maggie went off to a hotel further along the coast to begin the process of writing without distraction. The book's first half was completed within a week – with pencil and paper – and once back home, Maggie typed the chapter contents using her portable-manual typewriter, with cut and paste being a pair of scissors and a roll of sticky tape. Maggie's book was translated into Japanese, and when it came to the attention of a Tokyo businessman, he had a gut feeling that aromatherapy would one day be a great success throughout Japan. The first meeting, held in the UK, was the beginning of a twenty-three-year business relationship, with Maggie visiting Japan on five occasions. And in 1989, when Maggie delivered her first talks in Tokyo to attentive audiences, she was the very first speaker on the subject of aromatherapy in the whole of Japan; further talks were delivered in Kyoto and Osaka.

Meeting growers and distillers of aromatic plants involved considerable travel – mainly driving around the south of France – and Maggie, as a single mother, successfully juggled family and career for many years. Whilst visiting West Africa in the mid-1990s, Maggie became involved with a village project, where the cultivation of a fragrant plant was already being viewed as preferable to the existing farming of coffee and cocoa beans. Maggie wanted to help make a difference to the lives of the farmers by paying them a good price for every kilo of the aromatic oil, at a price agreed by the farmers, instead of the low price they were receiving for their coffee beans. Many families were too poor to have their children educated, as a village school will generally only allow a child to enrol in classes if the family can afford to buy a ruler, rubber, pencils, toothbrush and a bag to put them in. And also to pay for the teacher's time. Maggie invested considerable amounts of energy and funding, but sadly, had to abandon the dream of producing an excellent aromatic oil and helping twenty-five families, when the country fell into civil unrest followed by civil war, and the project had to be abandoned.

Checking BBC news for updates on the political situation in the West African country, Maggie accidentally came across news bulletins about hospital-acquired MRSA. Knowing that some essential oils were antibacterial, Maggie put together a blend of essential oils, tracked down a support group of people who had been badly affected by the disease, and set up a small trial with five volunteers within a few months. This private research eventually led to a five-year collaboration with the University of Brighton microbiology team and a series of successful in vitro trials with essential oils and strains of antibiotic-resistant bacteria. A scientific paper was published. But to bring that research to a broader audience, Maggie researched and wrote *Aromatherapy vs MRSA*, first published in 2011, a few months before her eldest daughter was diagnosed with aggressive cancer.

The loss of a child is tremendous, and many years passed before Maggie felt able to write again, but in 2019 she set up her own publishing company – to publish what was to have been her seventh book – *Ageing Healthily with Maggie*. The twelve-chapter book on various aspects of ageing healthily was put on hold when the coronavirus was predominantly taking the lives of the elderly; when nursing home residents were unable to have visits from their family members; when too many people were dying without being able to see their loved ones for a final hug.

So, from the early days of lockdown, Maggie has conceived the idea of a book that might offer some practical advice; has conducted a huge amount of research; and from the beginning of 2021 has written and published *Antiviral Aromatherapy*.

Books inspired by Maggie

Aromatherapy for Women
   – Harper Collins (Thorsons), 1985

Aromatherapy vs MRSA
   – Clarity Press, 2011

   – JKP (Singing Dragon), 2015

   – Hachette (Singing Dragon)

Antiviral Aromatherapy
   – Weaver Publishing, 2022

Ageing Healthily with Maggie
   – Weaver Publishing Ltd. To be confirmed

Book commissions

Essential Oils for Lovers
– Harper Collins, London & San Francisco, 1993

The Magic & Power of Lavender
(co-written with Monika Junneman)

– Schneelowe Verlag, Munich, Germany, 1989

The 14-Day Aromabeauty Plan
– Random House, London, 1994

Stress: The Aromatic Solution
– Hodder & Stoughton, London, 1996

Websites

www.weaver-publishing.com

www.maggietisserand.com

www.antiviralaromatherapy.blog

Maggie would love to hear from you but is unable to give personal medical advice.

You can message Maggie via any of the above websites.